# Satisfied

Baking with Whole Grain Goodness

Annette Reeder

*I will abundantly bless her provision;*
*I will satisfy her needy with bread.*
Psalm 132:15

Copyright © 2017, 2022. Designed Publishing
The Biblical Nutritionist, Annette Reeder. All rights reserved.
The Biblical Nutritionist, Glen Allen, VA 23060
TheBiblicalNutritionist.com

Information contained in *Satisfied, Baking with Whole Grain Goodness* is educational and merely offers nutritional support. To the knowledge of the editors and author the FDA has not approved this writing for any spiritual or physical benefit. This means you are putting your life in God's hands by applying Scripture to health. For physical diseases such as diabetes consult with a physician before altering the government designed eating plan.

No part of this publication may be reproduced, stored in a retrieval system, or transmitted in any way by any means-electronic or mechanical, photocopy, recording or otherwise-without prior permission of the copyrights holder, except as permitted by USA copyright law.

ISBN: 978-0-9853969-7-8

Library of Congress Control Number: 2017907964

Cover photograph by Stacey Burton

My heartfelt thanks go to the following friends for
their editing, cooking and photography.
It is their contributions that make this a beautiful book.

Kathy Barnes
Karen Moore
Tina Word
Mollie Reeder
Stacey Burton
Darlene Swanson
Wendy Hale

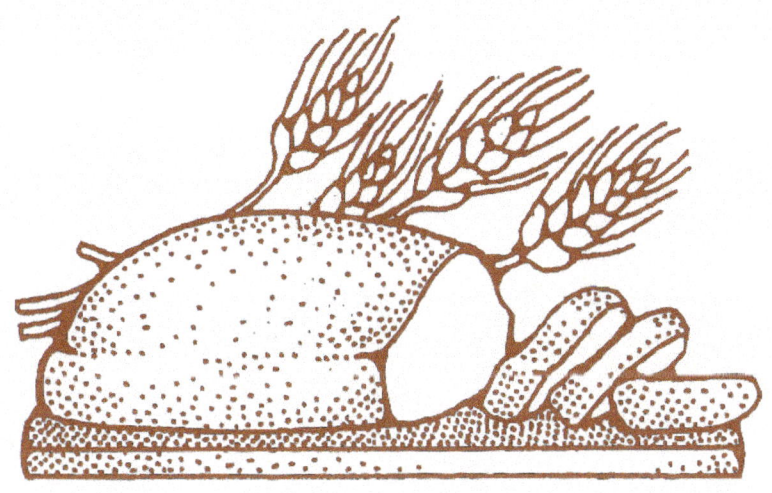

*I will abundantly bless her provision;*
*I will satisfy her needy with bread.*
Psalm 132:15

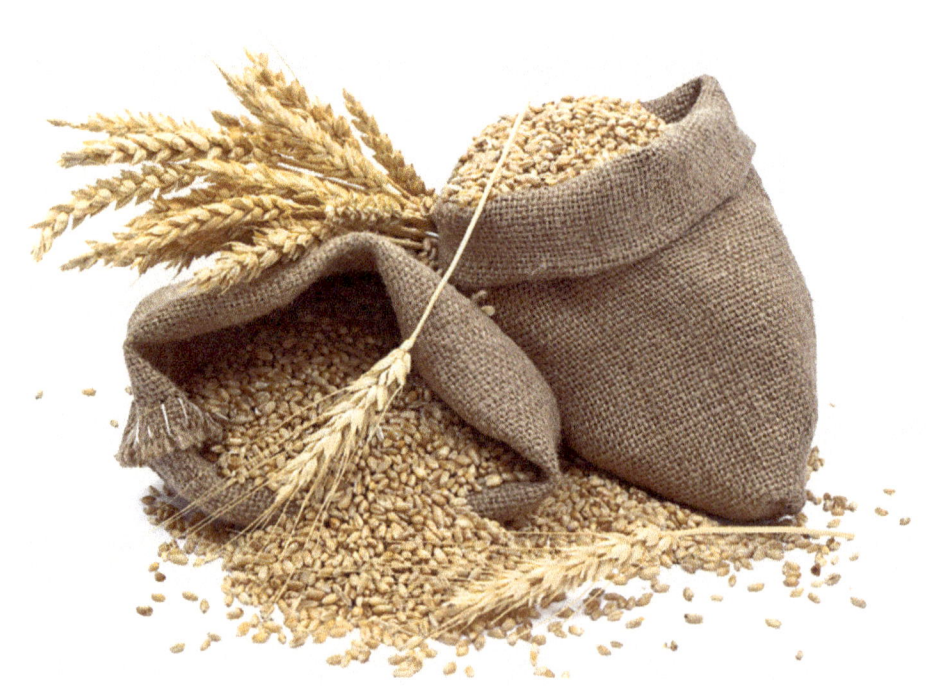

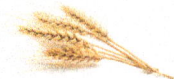

# Contents

Will the Real Bread Please Rise? . . . . . . . . . . . . . . . . . . . . . . . ix
Real Bread . . . . . . . . . . . . . . . . . . . . . . . . . . . . . . . . . . . . . 1
Grains—Goodness and Fiber . . . . . . . . . . . . . . . . . . . . . . . . 5
Whole Grains . . . . . . . . . . . . . . . . . . . . . . . . . . . . . . . . . . . 5
Grains of Value . . . . . . . . . . . . . . . . . . . . . . . . . . . . . . . . . . 6
History of White Flour . . . . . . . . . . . . . . . . . . . . . . . . . . . . 13
    Loss of Nutrients in White Flour . . . . . . . . . . . . . . . . . . . 16
Fiber Mystery Unfolded . . . . . . . . . . . . . . . . . . . . . . . . . . . 19
Fiber Facts . . . . . . . . . . . . . . . . . . . . . . . . . . . . . . . . . . . . . 23
    Two Types of Fiber . . . . . . . . . . . . . . . . . . . . . . . . . . . . 24
    How Much? . . . . . . . . . . . . . . . . . . . . . . . . . . . . . . . . 24
Getting Started Making Bread . . . . . . . . . . . . . . . . . . . . . . . 27
    Cost of Bread Savings . . . . . . . . . . . . . . . . . . . . . . . . . . 29
    The Perfect Mixer . . . . . . . . . . . . . . . . . . . . . . . . . . . . . 32

## Recipes

Classic Breads . . . . . . . . . . . . . . . . . . . . . . . . . . . . . . . . . . 37
    Whole Wheat Honey Bread (5 loaves) . . . . . . . . . . . . . . . 37
    Whole Wheat Honey Bread . . . . . . . . . . . . . . . . . . . . . . 39
    Honey Molasses Bread . . . . . . . . . . . . . . . . . . . . . . . . . 42
    Challah Prayer Bread . . . . . . . . . . . . . . . . . . . . . . . . . . 43

Stuffed ~ Rolled ~ Shaped Breads . . . . . . . . . . . . . . . . . . . . 45
    Hamburger Buns . . . . . . . . . . . . . . . . . . . . . . . . . . . . . 46

*Satisfied*

    Family Sandwich . . . . . . . . . . . . . . . . . . . . . . . . . . . . . . . . 47
    Feta-Spinach Bread . . . . . . . . . . . . . . . . . . . . . . . . . . . . . . . 48
    Cinnamon Bread . . . . . . . . . . . . . . . . . . . . . . . . . . . . . . . . . 50
    Garlic Herb Bread . . . . . . . . . . . . . . . . . . . . . . . . . . . . . . . . 51
    Sausage Cheese Bread. . . . . . . . . . . . . . . . . . . . . . . . . . . . . . 51
    Cheese Bread . . . . . . . . . . . . . . . . . . . . . . . . . . . . . . . . . . . 51
    Braided Apple Cinnamon . . . . . . . . . . . . . . . . . . . . . . . . . . . 52
    Spinach-Cheese French Bread . . . . . . . . . . . . . . . . . . . . . . . . 53
    Spinach Cheese Stromboli . . . . . . . . . . . . . . . . . . . . . . . . . . 54
    Stuffed Reuben Bread. . . . . . . . . . . . . . . . . . . . . . . . . . . . . . 54
    Turkey Stromboli . . . . . . . . . . . . . . . . . . . . . . . . . . . . . . . . . 55
    Ranch Pizza Pinwheels . . . . . . . . . . . . . . . . . . . . . . . . . . . . . 55
    Italian Bread . . . . . . . . . . . . . . . . . . . . . . . . . . . . . . . . . . . . 56
    Garlic Knots . . . . . . . . . . . . . . . . . . . . . . . . . . . . . . . . . . . . 57
    Cinnamon Croutons . . . . . . . . . . . . . . . . . . . . . . . . . . . . . . 58
    Garlic Croutons . . . . . . . . . . . . . . . . . . . . . . . . . . . . . . . . . . 58

Better Butters . . . . . . . . . . . . . . . . . . . . . . . . . . . . . . . . . . . . . . 60
    Cinnamon Butter . . . . . . . . . . . . . . . . . . . . . . . . . . . . . . . . 60
    Herbed Butter . . . . . . . . . . . . . . . . . . . . . . . . . . . . . . . . . . . 60
    Honey Butter . . . . . . . . . . . . . . . . . . . . . . . . . . . . . . . . . . . 60
    Lemon Butter. . . . . . . . . . . . . . . . . . . . . . . . . . . . . . . . . . . . 61
    Pecan Butter . . . . . . . . . . . . . . . . . . . . . . . . . . . . . . . . . . . . 61
    Strawberry Butter . . . . . . . . . . . . . . . . . . . . . . . . . . . . . . . . 61

Specialty Grains . . . . . . . . . . . . . . . . . . . . . . . . . . . . . . . . . . . . 62
    Easy Nutritious Pancakes GF . . . . . . . . . . . . . . . . . . . . . . . . . 62
    Family Table Talk . . . . . . . . . . . . . . . . . . . . . . . . . . . . . . . . . 63
    Spelt Crust Pizza . . . . . . . . . . . . . . . . . . . . . . . . . . . . . . . . . 64
    Cornbread . . . . . . . . . . . . . . . . . . . . . . . . . . . . . . . . . . . . . 66
    Ezekiel Grains . . . . . . . . . . . . . . . . . . . . . . . . . . . . . . . . . . . 67
    Russian Black Rye Bread . . . . . . . . . . . . . . . . . . . . . . . . . . . . 68

Holiday Favorites . . . . . . . . . . . . . . . . . . . . . . . . . . . . . . . . . . . 70
    Almond Raspberry Cheese Bread . . . . . . . . . . . . . . . . . . . . . . 70
    Cream Cheese Filling . . . . . . . . . . . . . . . . . . . . . . . . . . . . . . 70
    Apple Pie French Toast . . . . . . . . . . . . . . . . . . . . . . . . . . . . . 72

Cranberry Quinoa Scones . . . . . . . . . . . . . . . . . . . . . . . . . 73
Cranberry Wreaths . . . . . . . . . . . . . . . . . . . . . . . . . . . . . 74
Cranberry Filling . . . . . . . . . . . . . . . . . . . . . . . . . . . . . . 74
Cream Cheese Pumpkin Muffins . . . . . . . . . . . . . . . . . . . . 75
Easter Egg Nest Bread . . . . . . . . . . . . . . . . . . . . . . . . . . . 77
Pumpkin Bread Pudding . . . . . . . . . . . . . . . . . . . . . . . . . 79
Spicy Holiday Orange-Cranberry Bread . . . . . . . . . . . . . . . . 80
Sweet Potato Biscuits . . . . . . . . . . . . . . . . . . . . . . . . . . . 81

My Kitchen Prayer for You. . . . . . . . . . . . . . . . . . . . . . . . . . . . 83
About the author, Annette Reeder . . . . . . . . . . . . . . . . . . . . . . . 83
Bosch Attachments . . . . . . . . . . . . . . . . . . . . . . . . . . . . . . . 84
12 Tips For Perfect Bread . . . . . . . . . . . . . . . . . . . . . . . . . . . 87
Ingredients to Know. . . . . . . . . . . . . . . . . . . . . . . . . . . . . . . 89
    Bread Cooking Helps. . . . . . . . . . . . . . . . . . . . . . . . . . 92
(Endnotes). . . . . . . . . . . . . . . . . . . . . . . . . . . . . . . . . . . . . 93

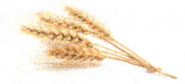

# Will the Real Bread Please Rise?

THERE IS CONFUSION IN THE hopper. Bread created for nourishment, fellowship, and spiritual awareness has become a topic of argument, upset, and all-out war. What has happened to cause delicious satisfying foods to become so confusing?

I still remember visiting my grandmother at the century family farm. She would carry a hot loaf of bread to the table using her well-worn apron as the pot holder. There would be a rush to get to the butter crock first and then to eagerly bite in to this warm delight. The thick slices and crunchy crust made it a treasured memory. No store bread could compete with Grandma's baked goodness. As we all enjoyed this buttered delight there would be three to four generations sitting around the old farm table sharing stories of the good ole days.

 For many people bread can conjure memories just like this.

Yet for other people, especially in today's culture, bread can bring thoughts of upset stomachs, toppling over waistlines, and lethargy.

What changed?

## Satisfied

I am glad you picked up this book. In it you will find the answer to that question plus many more. After I have calmed your anxiety about bread we will learn the basics of making and tasting *real* bread.

I still remember attending my first real bread class facilitated by my friend, Kim. Her bread was so rich and satisfying. Her encouragement was inspiring. Other teachings from Sue Becker have formed the foundation of my journey. Their combined inspiration to get back in Scriptures, eat real food, and delight in the Lord has transformed my life.

It is my prayer that this same revelation will convert your life. I pray your Spiritual and physical eyes are opened and your body is satisfied.

Enjoy God's goodness and be SATISFIED.

Baking Blessings,

*Annette Reeder*

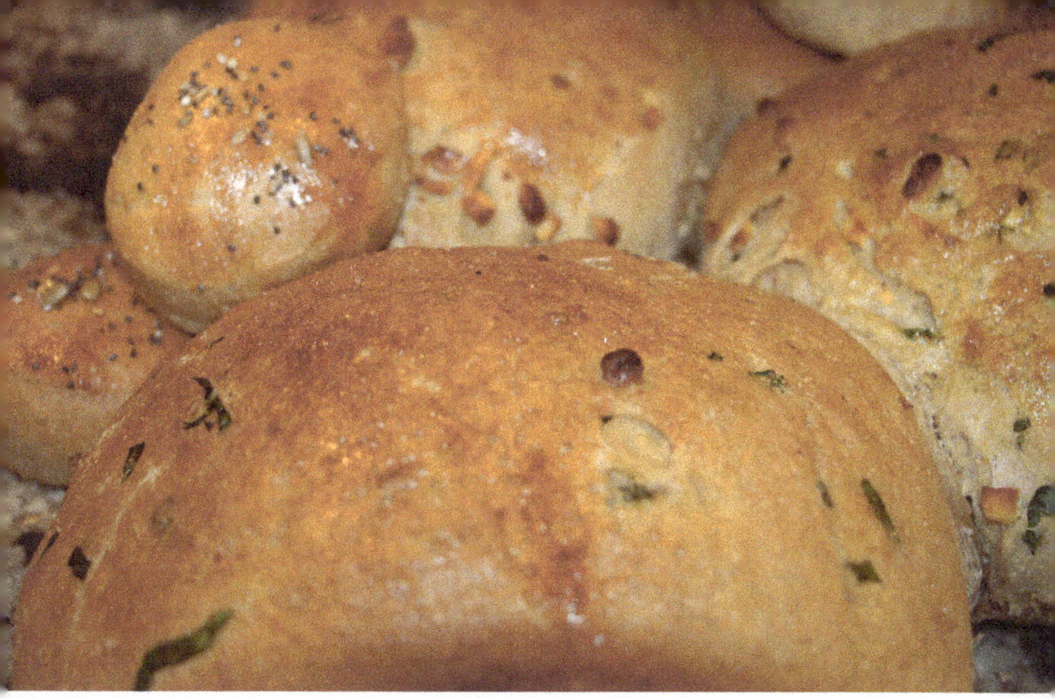

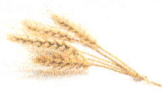

# Real Bread

*Why do you spend your money for what is not bread and your wages for what does not satisfy? Listen carefully to Me, and eat what is good, and delight yourself in abundance.*
Isaiah 55:2

*Give us this day our daily bread.*
Matthew 6:11

*And they were continually devoting themselves to the apostles teaching, and to fellowship, to the breaking of bread and to prayer.*
Acts 2:42

# Satisfied

*And day by day continuing with one mind in the temple, and breaking bread from house to house, they were taking their meals together with gladness and sincerity of heart.*
Acts 2:46

*I will abundantly bless her provision;
I will satisfy her needy with bread.*
Psalms 132:15

These verses illustrate the importance of bread. Jesus loved having others break bread with Him. Those were real times of blessing, intimacy, and revelation. Jesus broke bread with those on the road to Emmaus and their spiritual eyes were opened to know him. He broke bread with the disciples at the Passover and revealed the meaning of His death. After His resurrection, Jesus broke bread with the disciples and fellowshipped with them as they had breakfast together by the sea. In the book of Revelation, Jesus invited the lukewarm Christians to break bread with Him and allow their hearts to be rekindled by the fire of his love.

Breaking bread with Jesus means that we come and partake of who He is, enjoy His company and are nurtured by His presence. It means intimacy and communion. It means fellowship and the sharing of our hearts with His. Jesus never intended for us to break bread with Him occasionally; He intended us to break bread with Him on a daily basis.

He is the daily bread for which our soul should hunger.

He is the bread by which our spirits grow.

He is the bread that makes our hearts thrive.

He is the bread that brings us nourishment and sustains us through every step of the journey.

Come taste and see that the Lord is good. There is nothing more satisfying than partaking of the "bread of Life" which is our Lord.[1]

Further, the bread referred to in these verses is the daily bread of knowing Jesus as Lord. These verses also refer to the health value of making and eating bread daily. God designed the wheat kernel, as well as other grains to perfectly store the nutrients within. Once broken open, as in milling, the nutrients immediately begin to oxidize. Within about 72 hours 90% of over 30 nutrients are virtually gone.

This book along with other books written by Annette Reeder explain the dire story of wheat and the distancing that has taken place from God's plan to Satan's deception.

Since we have turned over the responsibility of preparing our bread daily to the manufacturers, we have also turned over to them our health. The resulting consequences are overwhelming.

God has given each of us the responsibility to prepare healthy meals for our family. Healthy meals include the best *real* bread. It is time to reclaim the health of our families and assume the role as their personal nutritionist.

Then we all enjoy the Real Bread.

---

1  Words originally written by Roy Lessin, not full quote.

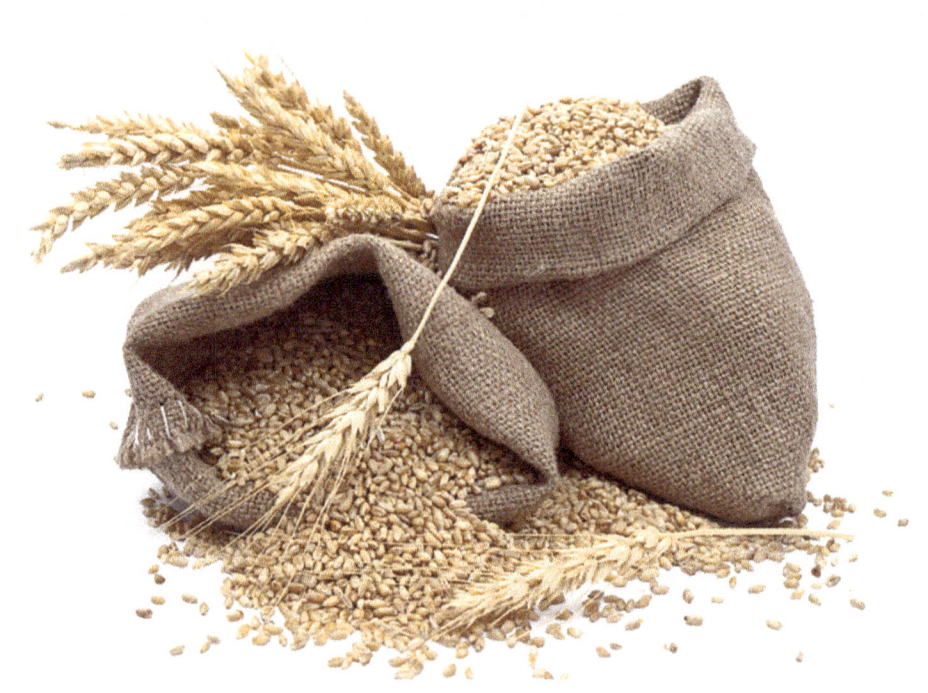

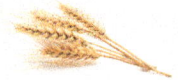

# Grains—Goodness and Fiber

*With the finest of wheat...*
Deuteronomy 32:14

## Whole Grains

Warm, fresh baked bread is the true taste of the goodness of grains. Nothing compares to this satisfying taste and the health-promoting abilities of fresh whole wheat bread. If we want to eat the foods Jesus ate, then whole grains belong on the table.

When someone first told me that I needed to mill my own wheat and make my own bread, all I could picture was a horse walking around a grind stone in my backyard. My neighbors would definitely disagree with that choice. Fortunately, today, we have the simple design of the Mock Mill to mill any grain, bean, or legume into fresh, satisfying, and nutritious flour.

Breads in the market have come far from God's original design. Today, the white flour used in over 99% of store purchased and restaurant served bread works the same as white sugar in the body. White flour has been robbed of its color, taste, smell and nutrients. Twenty-six nutrients plus the bran have been removed from wheat to produce white flour. Five of the removed nutrients are then returned (in a synthetic form) to produce "enriched" flour. This is the opposite of the Robin Hood effect!

Replacing white flour with freshly milled whole grain flours is a tremendous step in nutritional improvement. Freshly-milled flours have all of the natural oils and nutrients of the grain still intact. To retain the nutrients once the grain is ground into flour by a flour mill, the flour can be placed in the refrigerator or freezer for up to one month before the natural oils go rancid. If the freshly-ground flour is left at room temperature, the natural oils will go rancid within forty-eight hours. After that time, the wheat germ, containing ninety percent of the nutrients, is also rancid. "Rancid" basically means that the food item has spoiled and often will smell bad. Eating rancid or spoiled food has obvious consequences, the least of which is increased toxicity to the body.

Once the bread is baked within 12 hours of milling the nutrients are preserved.

Invest in your health and make smart choices. Whole grains add to your health. Processed, enriched, and fortified grains steal away your health. I guarantee you will be satisfied.

*Give us each day our daily bread.*
Luke 11:3

## Grains of Value

Journey through the field and tempt your taste with these grains of value:

### *Amaranth*

This poppy-seed sized grain, a botanical cousin to quinoa, has been a revered crop of the ancient Incas and Aztecs. It has a nutty and somewhat sweet flavor. It works best where a cohesive texture is desirable, as in spoon breads, casseroles, loaves, or hot cereals. Leftover cooked amaranth can be added in small quantities to muffins or quick breads.

## Barley

Barley is a short, stubby kernel with a hard outer shell. Pearled barley has the outer layer removed. Barley flour makes excellent pie crusts and cookies. It also mixes well with rice flour. It is the whitest of the whole grain flours and has a mild taste. It has no gluten and cannot be used with yeast.

## Buckwheat

Buckwheat is not related to wheat and is in the grass family. Buckwheat groats are most often used as the basis for kasha. The flour is more strongly flavored than many other flours and most often used in pancakes, waffles, and quick breads. Light colored and textured buckwheat flour can be made by placing hulled buckwheat groats in a blender and blending them into flour.

## Cornmeal

Made from corn and popcorn, cornmeal is used primarily in cornbread, polenta, and mush. Only use organic corn due to the high percentage of GMO corn grown.

## Einkorn

Einkorn is the earliest form of cultivated wheat, allegedly found in the tombs of ancient Egypt. It is unique in flavor, nutritional benefits and genetic makeup. Where modern wheat has 42 chromosomes, Einkorn has only 14. Einkorn is about 50% higher in protein than modern wheat yet its gluten structure makes it tolerable by some people with wheat sensitivities. Einkorn has 25% more riboflavin (vitamin B2 which stimulates the metabolism and assists in the digestion and absorption of fats, carbohydrates and proteins) than modern wheat. It also has higher beta carotene, lutein, and vitamin A. Einkorn is also a great source of minerals including zinc, manganese, potassium, phosphorus, and iron. Einkorn bakes similar to spelt.

## *Emmer wheat*

Emmer is one of the three hulled wheats known in Italy as farro. Its main use is for human food, though it is also used for animal feed. In recent years, farro has been enjoying a resurgence in popularity among gourmets and the health-conscious, who sing the grain's praises for its high nutritional value and adore the hearty, flavorful taste of the "Pharaoh's Wheat". Rich in fiber, protein, magnesium, and vitamins, emmer contributes to a complete protein diet when combined with legumes, making Emmer grains and pastas ideal for vegetarians (or for anyone simply looking for a plant-based high-protein food source). [1]

## *Kamut*

A relative of durum of wheat, kamut is Egyptian wheat. Kamut can sometimes be used in place of wheat for those with wheat allergies. It produces excellent breads, pastas, and other baked goods. It has a light, slightly-buttery flavor and a golden color.

## *Millet*

Millet was a staple food in many countries before the use of rice. It has a high-quality protein and is rich in calcium, iron, and potassium. It is also very easy to digest. It is often used as a morning cereal or in soups, stews, casseroles, stuffing, and puddings. Millet flour tends to be heavy and bland in flavor. Oven temperatures should be reduced by twenty-five degrees for millet flour products.

## *Oats*

Oats are an ideal cold-weather crop. They are second to amaranth and quinoa in protein, and rich in calcium, phosphorus, and iron. Since they have a slightly higher fat content, they produce a sense of warmness. Oat flour works well with cookies and pie crusts. Oat flour can be made by placing rolled or quick oats in the blender and blending until it is flour-like. Whole groats can be eaten uncooked for a chewy snack. My friend, Joyce Rogers, says the secret to her bread is adding 1 cup oat flour to the mix of wheat flour. This makes softer, richer flavored bread.

## *Pumpernickel*

True pumpernickel is coarsely ground rye flour. Most commercial pumpernickel breads have a white flour base with added rye flour for color and flavor.

## *Quinoa*

Traditionally grown in the Andes, the quinoa plant bears tan grains about the size of sesame seeds. Quinoa is similar to amaranth nutritionally; it yields a fluffier texture with a distinct flavor. Quinoa flour has a stronger flavor and is best mixed with other flours. Quinoa is a great replacement for rice in your regular dishes. See the *Healthy Treasures Cookbook* for delicious recipe options.

## *Rice*

Quickly becoming the most popular grain due to the rise in gluten intolerance, rice is mostly thought of in the varieties of white and brown. This is far from reality since rice comes in 18,000 different varieties. Even brown rice comes in seven different bran colors such as: white, light brown, speckled brown, brown, red, variable purple, and purple (black).

The design of rice is the same as wheat. It has the outer covering known as the bran which includes the nutrients of fiber, vitamin B, minerals, and protein. The second part is the endosperm which includes the carbohydrates and more protein and vitamin B. Finally, the germ has the highest amount of vitamins, minerals and phytonutrients. With all these nutrients rice can easily move from the side dish to the main course. It is in itself a complete protein with all amino acids present.

## Rice and Rice Flour

Flour made from brown rice can be gritty in texture and taste, but it is excellent for thickening gravies and sauces. Baked products made only from rice flour tend to be crumbly. Brown rice flour works very well when mixed with barley flour.

*All brown rice flour should be stored in the refrigerator to preserve the oil in the bran.

## Spelt

Spelt is believed to be among the most ancient of cultivated wheats. It is higher in fiber and protein than wheat and is easily digested. Spelt is favored by many people with wheat and gluten sensitivities since it is more tolerated. It has a nutty aroma and flavor. The gluten content is more fragile than wheat, so it should be kneaded less in yeast recipes.

## Triticale

A hybrid grain that is a cross between wheat and rye. It imparts a very mild rye flavor to baked goods.

## Storage of Grains

Whole grains should be kept in airtight containers in cool, dry places. They will last this way for a year or more. Placing a few bay leaves on top can help keep the grains bug free. If the grains are to be kept for a longer period of time, they should be kept in a five-gallon bucket with a "gamma-lid" for easy access. Five-gallon buckets can be purchased at local hardware stores, and gamma lids can be ordered from internet outlets. Some people have even acquired good icing containers from bakeries to use. These work perfectly for grains, beans, and other dry goods. Ask nicely and you may get one or more for free.

## *Cooking Suggestions*

To dry roast, simply add the grain to an ungreased pan and place it over medium heat. Shake or stir the pan continuously for three to six minutes. Remove the pan from the heat before the grains turn too dark and start to burn.

When cooking grains, you may substitute chicken, beef, or vegetable stock for half or all of the water called for in the recipe. As a rule, I suggest replacing no more than half of the water with stock so that the delicate flavor of the grains is allowed to shine through. I also suggest using a low-sodium stock if you buy it canned—the full-strength commercial stocks are extremely salty.

## Basic Recipe for Grains (makes 3 cups)

This recipe works fine for quinoa, millet, barley, and coarse-grain bulgur. See chart below for cooking times.

- 1 cup quinoa, millet, barley, or coarse-grain bulgur
- 6 cups water
- 1 teaspoon kosher salt

Rinse grain in a colander. Bring the water and salt to a simmer. Add grain and reduce heat to a steady simmer. Cook for the times shown in the chart below. Pour into a sieve or fine colander and let drain for 10 minutes. Fluff with a fork and serve.

## Cooking times for basic grains:

The cooking times below are to be used with the Basic Recipe for Grains (above).

- Quinoa: 10 minutes
- Millet: 12 minutes
- Pearl barley: 45 minutes
- Coarse bulgur: 12 minutes, remove from heat, let sit for 5 minutes, then drain.

This basic recipe for grains is an unlimited addition to any meal, breakfast to dinner. Chopped fruit and honey makes these grains perfect for an energizing breakfast. Add nuts, herbs, and veggies for a unique twist on salads, or to soups and stews for a texture and flavor boost.

The possibilities are endless. In fact, there are a number of recipes using these and other whole grains in my *Healthy Treasures Cookbook*.

I have a fun challenge for you. Cook some grains using the recipe above, and be creative with a current favorite dish by adding one of the grains. Or create a new dish and share your nutritional secret with others in the spirit of hospitality and fellowship. I would love to hear of your grain adventures Visit us at: TheBiblicalNutritionist.com.

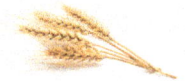

# History of White Flour

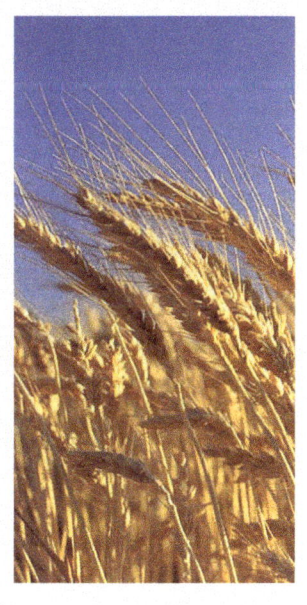

WARM ROLLS, HOT BISCUITS, HEARTY pancakes—great tasting bread has been in our diets since the beginning. Then along came the "low carb" diets giving bread a bad name. What is the real truth? Let's look at how the wheat grain contributes to good health while white flour deteriorates our health.

The wheat kernel was created, as well as other grains, to be stored perfectly packed with abundant nutrients. It is like a child who has their suitcase continually packed ready to go to Disney World. Once the kernel is broken by milling, the nutrients begin to oxidize. Within about 72 hours over 90% of all nutrients are virtually gone. The absence of these nutrients and the bulk of the fiber is the cause of suffering from health problems such as the ones listed on the Fiber Analysis (see pages 19–20).

When the wheat kernels are milled into white flour, the bran and the germ are removed. Only the endosperm remains in white flour. The removal of these nutrients is reflected on the next page. This process of removal allows the bleached white flour to be stored indefinitely.

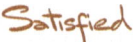

| Before | | Removed During Processing | | | After |
|---|---|---|---|---|---|
| Whole Grain | Bran | Middlings | Germ | Germ Oil | White Flour |
| Over 30 known nutrients | Insoluble fiber aids regularity | Balances blood sugar | Nutrient-rich for intestinal health | Highest vitamin E content of any food | Harmful pesticides, fungicides, bleaching & maturing agents and synthetic vitamins added. |
| Protective shell locks in nutrients | High in trace minerals | Helps maintain energy levels | Detoxifies blood | | |
| | Satisfies hunger quickly | | | | |

\*\* Any bread that can be displayed on a grocery store shelf longer than 3 days has had the vital nutrients removed or rancidity would occur. Rancidity causes bread to smell bad and mold.

## Common Additives and Chemicals Found in Processed Breads

L. Cysteine (dough conditioner): Amino acid derived from human hair, hog hair or duck feathers.

Mono and Diglycerides (emulsifiers): Common chemical additives to help prevent bread from becoming stale.

Potassium Bromate (maturing agent): banned in Europe, Australia, China, Brazil and Canada. Don't be fooled because the FDA labels it as safe.

Ammonium Sulfate (rising agent): Dangerous compound most often used as a fertilizer and also common in flame retardants.

Sodium Stearoyl Lactate (texture enhancer): May exacerbate digestive problems in those with lactose intolerance.

Calcium Propionate (preservative): Known to create allergic reactions, sleep problems, and restlessness in children.

## A Kernel of Truth

What has happened to the milling of wheat flour to make white flour is a good example of how we have been robbed of important nutrients that God created for our benefit. Some people refer to this as the "great grain robbery"!

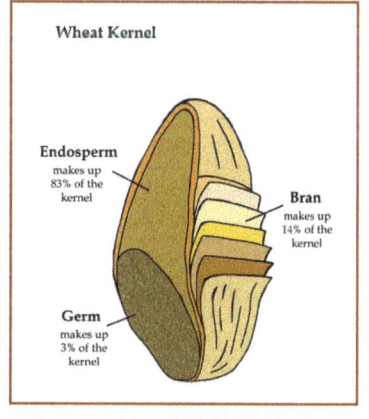

When the wheat kernels are milled into white flour, the bran and the germ are removed. Only the endosperm remains in white flour. The chart on pages 16-17 shows how much nutrient value is lost.

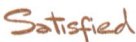

## Loss of Nutrients in White Flour

> **VITAMINS:**
>
> B-1, B-2, B-3, iron and folic acid are added to white flour in **synthetic** form

| WHOLE WHEAT FLOUR | LOSS IN WHITE FLOUR |
|---|---|
| Thiamine (B-1) | 77% |
| Riboflavin (B-2) | 67% |
| Niacin (B-3) | 81% |
| Pyridoxine (B-6) | 72% |
| Choline | 30% |
| Folic acid | 67% |
| Pantothenic acid | 50% |
| Vitamin E | 86% |
| Chromium | 40% |
| Manganese | 86% |
| Selenium | 16% |
| Zinc | 98% |
| Iron | 75% |
| Cobalt | 89% |
| Calcium | 60% |

| WHOLE WHEAT FLOUR | LOSS IN WHITE FLOUR |
|---|---|
| Sodium | 78% |
| Potassium | 77% |
| Magnesium | 85% |
| Phosphorus | 91% |
| Molybdenum | 48% |
| Copper | 68% |
| Fiber | 89% |

*Vitamins B-1, B-2, B-3, and iron are added to white flour in synthetic form by a process called "enrichment."

** Original source: Henry A. Schroeder, "Losses of Vitamins and Trace Minerals Resulting from Processing and Preservation of Foods," **American Journal of Clinical Nutrition** 241971); revalidated at www.ars.usda.gov/research/publications/publications.htm?seq.no_115=2-3150

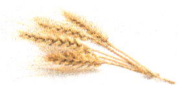

# Fiber Mystery Unfolded

## A Fiber Analysis

| INSOLUABLE FIBERS | SOLUABLE FIBERS |
|---|---|
| **Food Sources** | **Food Sources** |
| Bran of whole grains:<br>    wheat bran<br>    corn bran<br>    rice bran<br>    Legumes | Oats (bran)<br>Dried fruits<br>Apples, pears (flesh)<br>Membranes of oranges<br>Most vegetables<br>Seeds, Barley, Spelt |

| INSOLUABLE FIBERS | SOLUABLE FIBERS |
|---|---|
| Assists digestive regularity contributing to the prevention and regulation of:<br>    Appendicitis<br>    Colon cancer<br>    Constipation<br>    Crohn's disease<br>    Diverticular disease<br>    Hemorrhoids<br>    Hiatal hernia<br>    Obesity<br>    Spastic colon<br>    Ulcerative colitis<br>    Varicose veins | Helps regulate appropriate blood sugar and cholesterol levels contributing to prevention and regulation of:<br>    Coronary heart disease<br>    Diabetes<br>    Gallstones<br>    High blood pressure<br>    Hypoglycemia |
| Cellulose is a form of fiber from the foods listed above that forms mucus in the intestine, destroying the parasite that causes irritable bowel syndrome. | Recent studies show that rice and barley bran lower cholesterol, perhaps not because of the fiber, but because of antioxidant properties in the oil of the grain. |

The appearance of the steel roller mill marked the end of fiber consumption as we knew it. The roller mill, invented in 1870, was a quick and inexpensive way to separate the white inner substance (low in nutrients) of the grain from the outer bran and germ, both of which contain most of the key nutrients and nearly all of the fiber in the grain.

It was ideal for marketing. Whole wheat was a pain. The bugs ate the bran, and the germ would spoil. The inner white substance (endosperm) was resistant to spoilage (read "long shelf life"), and even the bugs ignored it, for the most part.

The popularity of refined products took off like a rocket. In many parts of America, in a very short time, cereal-fiber intake dropped by ninety percent. At the same time, consumption of fiber, including whole grains, beans, fresh vegetables, and fresh fruits, dropped (by fifty percent since 1910).

About this same time, sugar refining methods also became more sophisticated, and sugar began to appear in our diets in large amounts. Sugar is an excellent preservative and is added to most canned vegetables. In 1900, the average sugar consumption was 29 pounds per person per year. Now it is 150 pounds per person per year, and among teenagers consumption is reaching even higher amounts.

As time has passed, more and more of the diet of western man has come to consist of sugar, fat, and white flour in various forms. Items such as ultra-refined breads, cereals, doughnuts, cakes, pies, cookies, instant potatoes, and white rice have become norms on American tables.

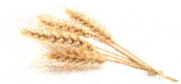

# Fiber Facts

*Earnestly desire the greater gifts, and
I show you a still more excellent way.*
1 Corinthians 12:31

IT WOULD BE INCOMPLETE TO study grains without understanding fiber and its role in health. Did you know the following facts about fiber?

- Fiber is the structural material that makes up all plants. It is not a nutrient; therefore, it is not absorbed into the bloodstream. It is resistant to digestion by secretions of the digestive tract; therefore, it passes through the body. In this passing, it has some remarkable effects on our health.

- Fiber decreases intestinal transit time, which moves food more quickly through the GI tract (fewer toxins build up).

- Fiber increases intestinal micro-flora benefit with a more favorable medium in which they thrive.

- An increased sense of fullness after eating fiber helps one eat less and enjoy it more.

- Increasing the daily intake of fiber by 10 grams decreases the risk of heart disease by 20 percent.

- By reducing harmful fat intake and increasing fiber intake, one can reduce the risk of colon cancer by 30 percent.

- Fiber acts like an ambulance driver, as it takes dead Candida out of the body to the morgue (toilet).

- Fiber results in increased energy, helps control weight, and really make a difference in blood profile. Your doctor will wonder what you have been doing when he sees your blood work.

## Two Types of Fiber

**Insoluble Fiber is** found in fruits and vegetables, wheat bran, whole grain cereals, whole wheat bread, nuts, and skins of fruits. Insoluble fiber plays an important role in bowel regularity. It absorbs and holds moisture, thereby producing larger stools and promoting regularity.

**Soluble Fiber is** found in fruits, nuts, legumes, plant seeds, and some vegetables (such as cabbage), and oat bran. Soluble fiber causes proper utilization of sugars and fats. It helps with diabetes, hypoglycemia, insulin resistance, cholesterol issues, and high blood pressure.

Good sources of both types of fiber are apples, wheat bran, whole grains, and dried fruits.

## How Much?

The National Cancer Institute recommends 25–30 grams of fiber per day. Others suggest 35–50 grams. Diabetics need over 50 grams daily. Research indicates that Americans eat approximately 8–12 grams of fiber per day.

Word of caution! Increase fiber slowly in your diet. Too much too quickly may produce digestive discomfort and unfavorable changes in daily bathroom schedules. Increasing fiber gradually and enjoying the positive consequences will give the added incentive to maintain recommended levels of fiber in the diet.

## *Low Fiber Diets Lead To*

1. Constipation
2. High cholesterol
3. Cancer
4. Diverticulitis
5. Appendicitis—Appendicitis can occur when a hard lump of constipated stool blocks the opening of the appendix and bowel bacteria multiply in the appendix.
6. Hemorrhoids
7. Varicose Veins
8. Hiatal Hernia
9. Irritable Bowel Syndrome
10. Gallstones
11. Diabetes
12. Increase in Toxins in Bloodstream
13. Weight Gain and Obesity

## *Important Benefits of Fiber*

1. Decreases likelihood of constipation. Fiber acts as a sponge, absorbing liquid, so that stools are softer and bulkier: therefore, they can pass through intestines more rapidly and easily.
2. Therefore, bowel disorders such as IBS, hemorrhoids, diverticulitis, cancer of the colon and rectum are reduced. In the US, 141,000 new cases of colon cancer are expected every year with 50,000 dying from this disease yearly. Do you want to be one of those statistics?
3. Lowers cholesterol and high blood pressure. Fiber latches onto the cholesterol in the bowel and prevents it from being reabsorbed into the bloodstream.
4. Researchers studied fiber intakes in twenty developed

*Satisfied*

countries. Japan ranked the highest in fiber intake and had the lowest rank in coronary heart disease, while the US ranked the lowest in fiber intake and the highest in coronary heart disease. Soluble fiber, such as that found in oats, fruits, legumes, and different gums, is best for lowering cholesterol.

5. Decreases possibility of varicose veins, hiatal hernias, and gallstones.
6. Improves control of diabetes. Insulin needs are reduced.
7. Protection from toxic products.
8. Weight reduction and control.
9. Anti-carcinogenic. Wheat bran bonds nitrate (cancer-causing chemical), making it unavailable to form cancer-causing nitrosamines. Fiber, like chlorophyll, may prevent carcinogens from entering cells.

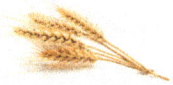

# Getting Started Making Bread

I am confident by now that this reading has piqued your interest in eating more fiber and baking bread. And if you have been blessed enough to enjoy the Bread making classes we teach then you have tasted the difference.

Are you ready to be satisfied? Let's get started!

The thought of buying tools and machines can be daunting but be comforted. This has been one of the best decisions I have ever made for the health of my family. My family gets the full nutritional impact when I make pancakes, muffins, breads and all recipes requiring whole grains from grains I milled myself!

We haven't even talked about the fun of milling dry beans to make a quick bean dip or hummus. This discovery opens a new door to entertainment and fellowship.

Depending on the method chosen for milling and baking there are a few items needed to get started. Listed here are the tools and equipment my baker friends and myself prefer. Visit our website at TheBiblicalNutritionist.com to purchase tools and equipment designed to bring healthy cooking back in style.

What you need to get started with mixer mixing:

- Bosch Universal: my favorite – preferred over Kitchen Aid
- Mock Mill (Much preferred over the Wondermill or Whisper Mill)
- 4 8-inch waffle weave or stainless steel loaf pans
- Yeast –vacuum packed professional yeast is most economical
- Real Salt – least processed brand of sea salt and loaded with trace minerals.
- Dough scraper- makes it fun and easy to work with dough
- Heavy duty bread bags (washable, reusable)
- Wheat: Hard Red, Hard White, Soft White (pastry flour), other options could be Spelt, Kamut, etc.
- Gamma Lid – tight sealing lid for years of protecting your wheat and your fingers.
- Optional Ingredients: Vital Wheat Gluten and Dough Enhancer

## *What you need to get started with a bread machine:*

- Mock Mill, Harvest Mill, Classic Nutrimill, or Nutrimill Plus
- Zojuirishi (programmable horizontal loaf)bread machine
- Package of yeast
- Real Salt
- Heavy duty bread bags
- Wheat

Baking with Whole Grain Goodness

## *What you need to get started with hand kneading:*

- Mock Mill
- Real Salt
- Heavy duty bread bags
- Package of yeast
- One dough scraper
- Wheat

## Cost of Bread Savings

| Ingredient | Weight | Total Ingredients Costs | Unit Cost | Amount Used | Total Batch Cost |
|---|---|---|---|---|---|
| Wheat | 25 lbs | $30.00 | 1.20 lb. | 5 lbs | $6.00 |
| Honey | 3 lbs | $20.00 | $6.66 lb. | 8 oz. | $3.33 |
| Oil | 48 oz. | $3.50 | .08 oz. | 5 oz. | .40 |
| Salt | 26 oz. | $1.00 | .04 oz. | 1 oz. | .04 |
| Yeast | 16 oz. | $4.00 | .25 oz. | .7 oz. | .20 |
| Dough enhancer | 16 oz. | $6.00 | .38 oz. | .6 oz. | .24 |
| Gluten | 27 oz. | $8.00 | .30 oz. | .7 oz. | .21 |
| Total | | $72.50 | | | $10.22 for 5 loaves |

Average loaf of healthy store bought bread in your area $ _____

Subtract $ _1.37_ (*this figure is total cost per loaf. Cost per loaf divided by the # of loaves)

Average Savings per loaf $ _____

Divide the cost of your Bosch by the average savings per loaf to figure out how many loaves you would need to make to pay for your Bosch $ _____

*Satisfied*

## 3 Nutrimills to choose from:

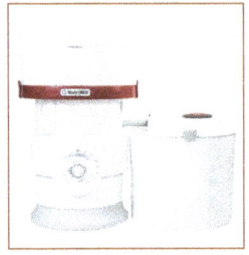
Nutrimill Plus

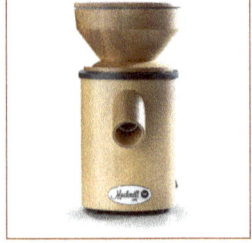
Mock Mill

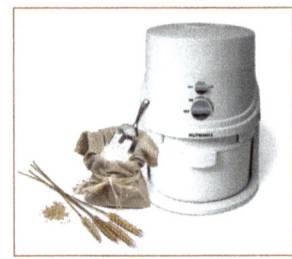
Nutrimill Classic

## Mock Mill Grain Mill

- Freshly milled flour on demand with the Mockmill. Discover the variety, flavor and energy in freshly milled grains.

- The Mock Mill has been a delightful change from my Nutrimill. The variety settings offer much more versatility from cracked grains to super fine flour. Plus the flour can be milled a second time for even finer flour.

- Easy to operate

- Simple to clean

- Easy and quick adjustment of the settings from very fine to coarse by rotating hopper

- Throughput of approximately 100 g (3.5 oz) of wheat / minute

- Sturdy industrial motor

- Milling mechanism consisting of corundum-ceramic milling stones

- Made in Germany

- 2-year warranty for commercial use

- 12-year warranty for private use

## Nutrimill Classic

This is my first mill and I used it for over 10 years. It is simple and efficient. If you visit my YouTube channel I share a comparison of mills and you can learn more. YouTube: The Biblical Nutritionist.

The NutriMill Classic allows you to grind up to 20 cups of flour at one time! Its grain hopper and flour bin are perfectly matched so you never have to worry about an overfilled mess. Convenient, powerful & fast: Just pour grain in the hopper, turn the NutriMill Classic on, and its powerful 10 amp, 1-¾ hp motor does the rest, quickly producing your choice of fine, medium, or coarse flour. The NutriMill Classic's impact grinding mechanism is self-cleaning, and it operates dust-free, so grinding grain won't mean extra housecleaning later. Its one-piece design, easy-grip handles, and lightweight make the NutriMill Classic easy to move.

## Nutrimill Plus

The versatile NutriMill Plus grinds up to 24 cups wheat (both hard and soft), oat groats (dehulled oats), spelt, kamut, triticale, rice, dry beans, lentils, dent (field) corn, popcorn, dried sweet corn, split peas, buckwheat, rye, barley, millet, quinoa, amaranth, teff, sorghum, dried mung beans, and soybeans. It will also grind dried just-sprouted grain. The NutriMill Plus isn't suitable for spices, herbs, oilseeds such as flax, chopped chestnuts, or fibrous materials. Grains and beans that have already been milled can't be milled again in any impact mill, including the NutriMill Plus. The NutriMill Plus is an outstanding machine for making a full range of flour and meal textures.

## The Perfect Mixer

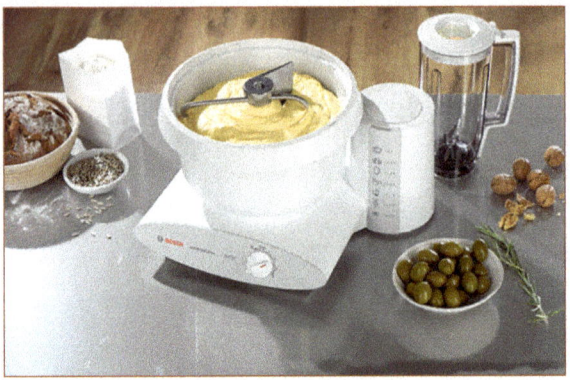

### *Bosch Universal Mixer*

**The Total Kitchen Center:** This Bosch Mixer is a complete kitchen center. It's the world's premier mixer and bread maker and in a single, exceptionally-engineered machine. Available attachments extend its range of abilities to include powerful blending, food processing, food grinding and more.

**Better Gluten Development:** The Bosch Universal Mixer has achieved its dedicated following among bread lovers not only because it lasts, but also because it *produces*. It makes better bread, faster and easier. Have 8 loaves piping hot fresh from your oven in 75 minutes from grinding wheat with this great machine.

**Mixing & Whipping:** The Bosch Mixer's whipping action is so energetic it will make a cup and a half of meringue from a single egg white.

**Optional Accessories** From food processing to making pasta, the Bosch Universal gives you the tools to do the job right. See our website to enjoy all the extras.

**The Warranty is Proof:** The Bosch mixer warranty backs up the claim that this is a better machine. The Bosch mixer motor and transmission are guaranteed for **3 full years!** To get equal warranty coverage from the competition, you'd have to buy three of their mixers.

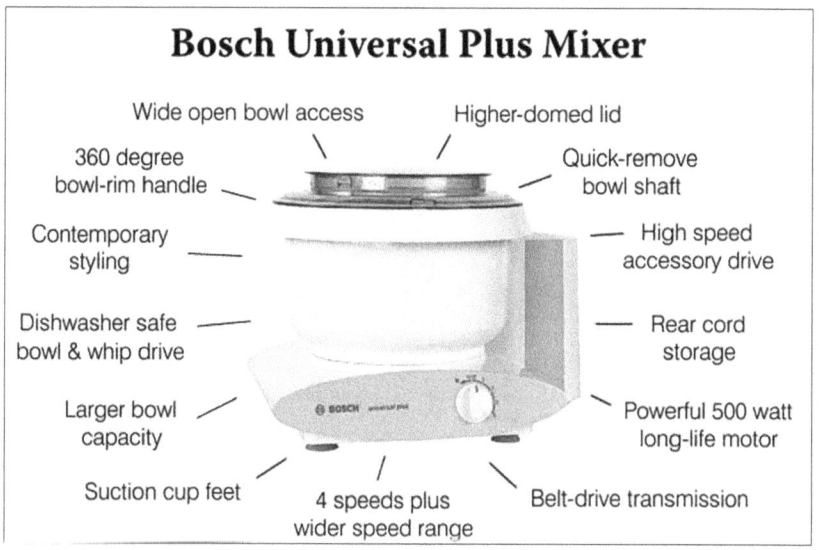

The newest model is the Bosch Universal Plus. Its 500 watt motor has a new design that extends motor life expectancy fourfold... and it was exceptionally long before. Just as importantly, the Bosch has a unique transmission that gets the motor's hard-turning torque to the bowl better than in other mixers. Other new features include suction cup feet, a larger, lockdown bowl with 360 degree handle, and a pop-out drive shaft for easy cleanup. Another speed was added, while expanding the speed range with a lower low gear and a higher high gear, still including the pulse feature. The distinct advantages of the Universal Plus over ordinary mixers are now greater than ever before.

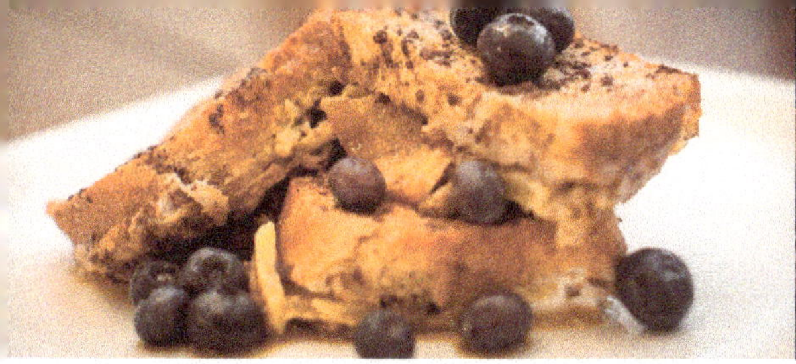

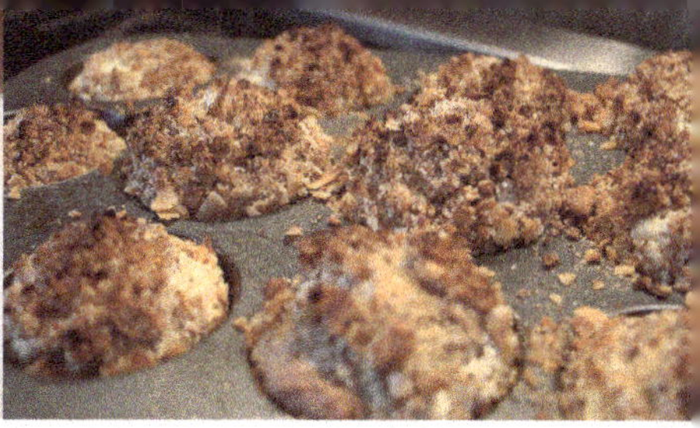

# Recipes

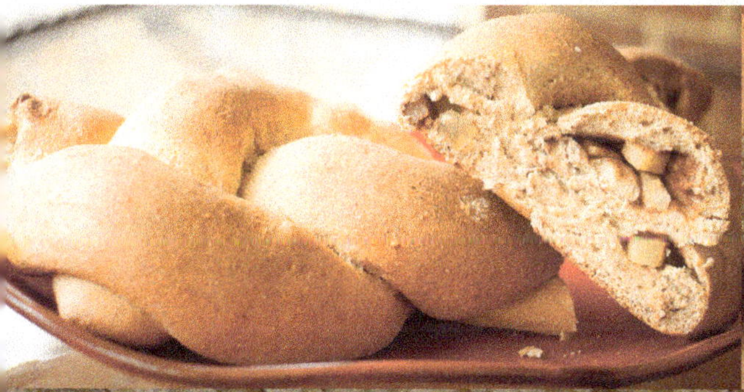

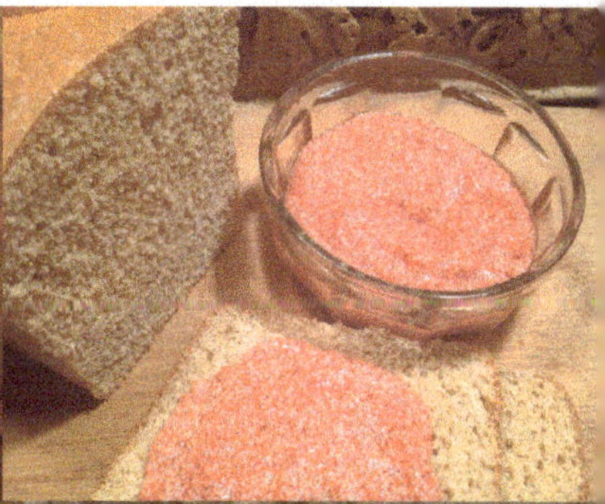

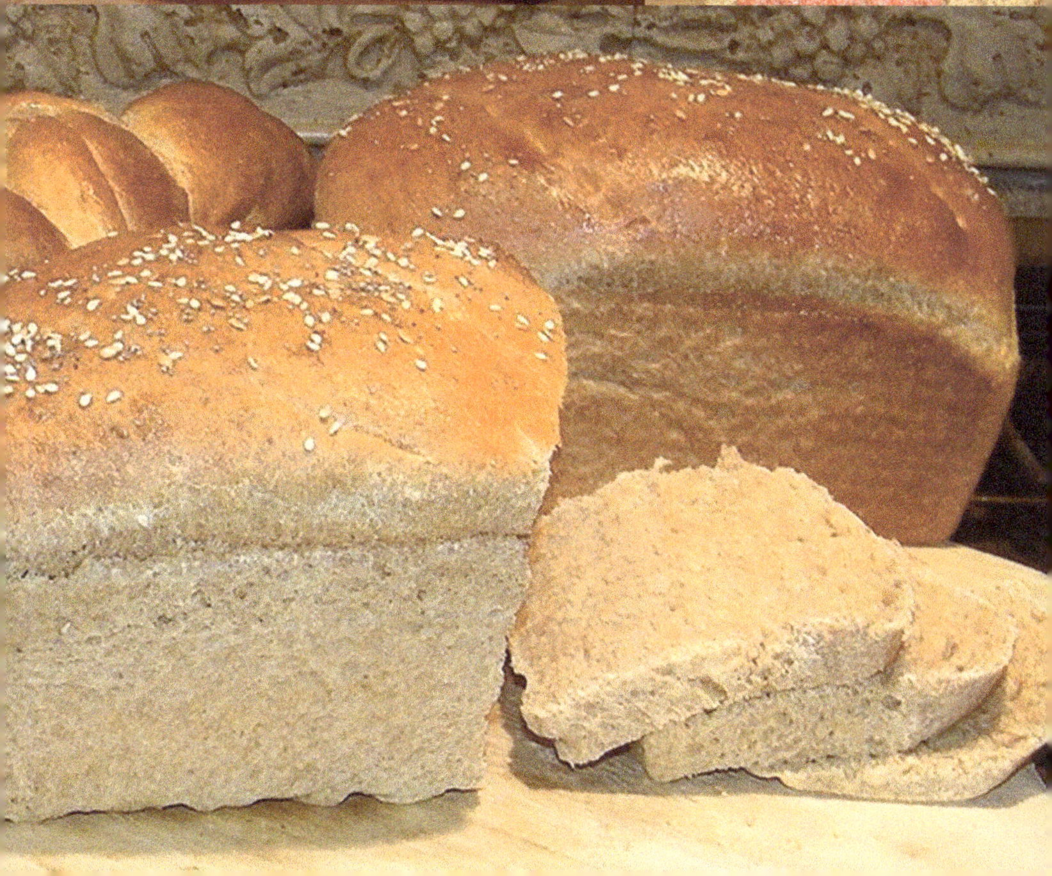

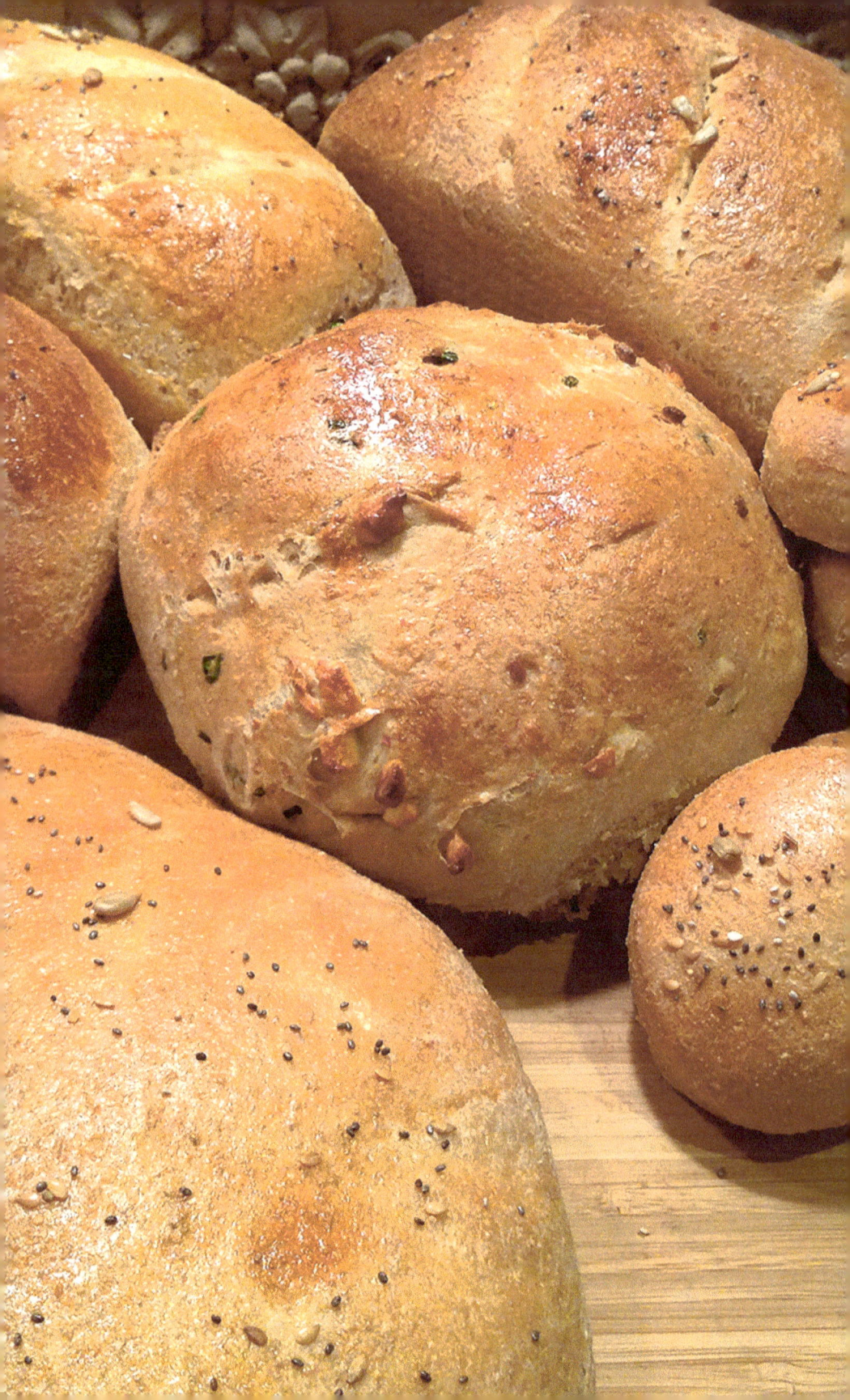

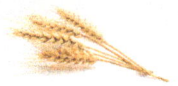

# Classic Breads

## Whole Wheat Honey Bread (5 loaves)

Mill 13 cups of grain – 19-21 cups of flour. Set aside.

| | |
|---|---|
| 6 | cups warm water |
| ¾ | cup olive oil |
| 1⅓ | cup honey |
| 4 | eggs |
| 4 | tablespoons yeast |
| 2 | tablespoons dough enhancer - optional |
| 4 | tablespoons lecithin – optional |

*To sponge means to let sit covered. As the yeast begins to consume the sugars the dough will rise and bubbles will appear. This can be considered the first rise.*

Mix the above ingredients plus 10 cups of the milled flour in the Bosch mixer until mixed. Then let sponge for 15 minutes.

### Next add:

1½   tablespoons gluten - optional
2     tablespoons salt
10-11 cups of flour

Mix in flour until the dough begins to pull away from the sides of the machine. Clean sides while mixing means there is enough flour. Let the machine knead the dough for 5-7 minutes. Remove the dough and shape into the loaf pans. Let rise for 30 minutes covered in a draft free place or until doubled in size.

Bake for 27 minutes at 350°F.

When making 5 loaves – don't think that is too much. Instead of thinking – pray "Lord, who do you want me to share this bread with?"

Ovens will vary with temperatures and times for baking. A dark golden color is perfect. To test the bread for doneness take the loaf out of the oven and remove from the pan. Thump the bottom. If you hear a hollow sound it is perfect.

## Bread Facts
According to historians 70 different kinds of bread were consumed in the first millennia BC.

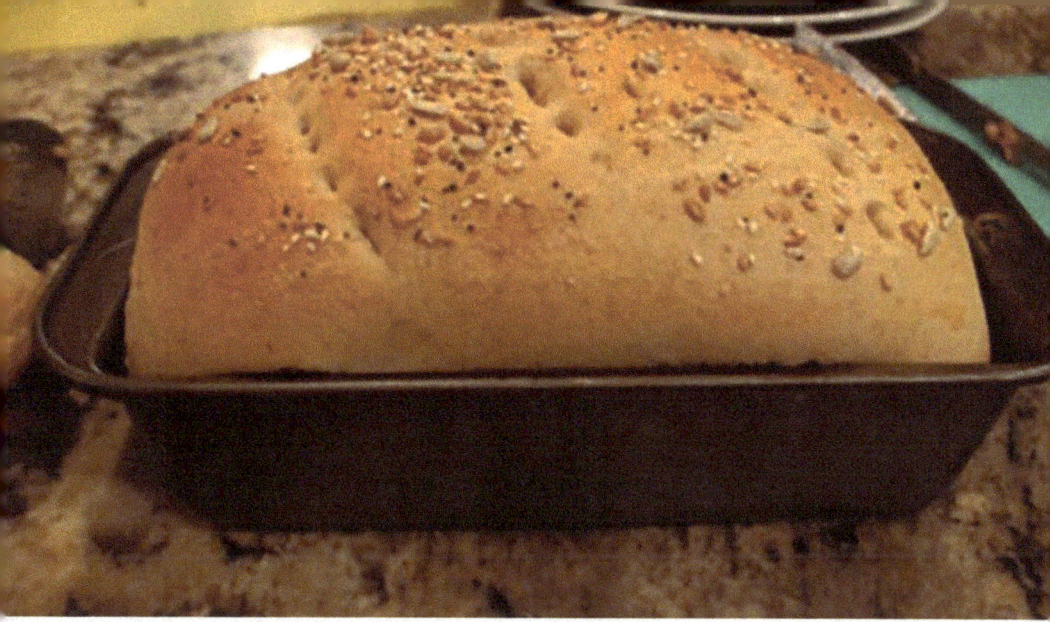

# Whole Wheat Honey Bread

## One Loaf Bread Machine Recipe

- 1½ cups hot water
- ⅓ cup olive oil
- ⅓ cup honey – less is ok
- 5 cups whole wheat flour – hard red or hard white
- 2 teaspoons salt
- 2 tablespoons lecithin – optional
- 2 tablespoons ground flax seed – optional
- 1 egg
- 1 tablespoon yeast

Place ingredients in your bread machine in the order given. Make sure paddles are in place first. Bake on the desired setting. My family's favorite bread recipe can be used for buns and rolls. Makes 20 rolls.

**Bread Machine:** Set the bread machine on dough cycle. Then when the cycle is finished, take the dough out of the bread machine and shape it into a prepared loaf pan. If the dough is a little sticky knead a small amount of flour into it as you shape it.

Place in a greased loaf pan. Let rise for approx. 40 minutes or until doubled in size.

Bake at 350°F for 27 minutes. Makes 2- one pound loaves or 1- two pound loaf.

**Bosch or Hand Mixing:** This recipe can be made with the Bosch mixer or by hand. Combine half the flour with the ingredients in the mixer and mix or stir for 2 minutes. Let sit for 15 minutes. Then add the remaining flour. After the remaining flour has been added keep the mixer kneading the dough for 7 minutes. The dough should pull away from the sides of the bowl. If it does not pull away add more flour in small amounts till it does.

After the kneading shape dough into the form you are baking and let rise for 30 minutes. After dough has risen to double its size bake for 27 minutes.

## Baking Notes

Converting recipes from refined white flour to whole grain flour is often a matter of trial and error. Many factors, such as the type of recipe, climate, and choice of texture when grinding, all play a part in the final results. Keep notes on how much flour used and whether more or less is needed next time. It may take a few attempts before you find just the right amount to suit your taste.

Choose flour texture (fine, medium or coarse) carefully. It affects the amount of flour needed and the final texture. Fine flour is good for cookies and pastries, but is not recommended for yeast bread. Instead choose a medium texture for bread flour. Coarse flour or meal is best for hot cereals or in small amounts to add crunch baked goods.

# Multi Grain Bread

2 Loaves

| | |
|---|---|
| 1 | tablespoon yeast |
| 6 | cups freshly milled wheat or spelt flour |
| 1 | cup oatmeal flour |
| 1 | teaspoon salt |
| ¼ | cup mixed seeds* |
| 2 | cups warm water |
| ⅔ | cup warm almond milk |
| 3 | tablespoons olive oil |
| 8 | tablespoons honey |
| 2 | eggs |

*In a sealable dry container mix seeds of all varieties such as sunflower seeds, pumpkin, poppy, amaranth, sesame seeds, chia, flax, millet and even oat flakes.*

*Keep handy in the freezer for adding into bread or muffins or as a decorative topping.*

Mix 5 cups of the flour with all ingredients in the Bosch mixer. Save the last cup of flour until after all ingredients are completely mixed. Add more flour until the sides of the bowl no longer have dough sticking to it. Once the dough is good and not sticking to the sides of the bowl as it mixes, let the Bosch knead the bread dough for 5-7 minutes.

Place bread dough in prepared bread pans ⅔ full. Cover with cloth and set in warm location to rise. When doubled bake for 25 minutes at 350° F.

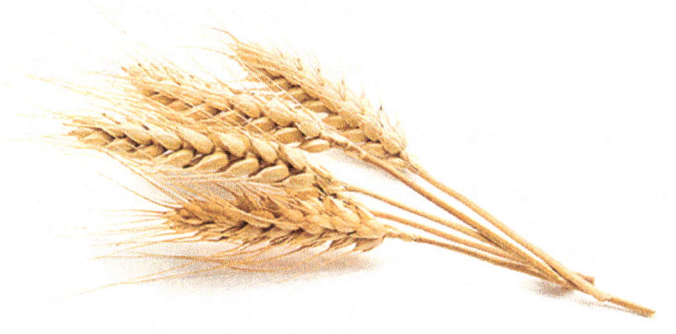

# Honey Molasses Bread

Makes 2 loaves.

Preheat oven to 375°F.

In Bosch Mixer with dough hook or by hand:

| | |
|---|---|
| 2 | cups warm water |
| ⅔ | cup warm almond milk |
| 3 | tablespoons oil |
| 1½ | teaspoon salt |
| 4 | tablespoons honey |
| 4 | tablespoons molasses |
| 2 | eggs |
| 1 | tablespoon gluten |
| 1 | teaspoon dough enhancer |
| 6 | cups freshly milled flour (spelt, einkorn and kamut are good options) |
| 1 | cup powdered rolled oats (oats pulsed in dry blender) |
| ⅔ | cups raisins |
| 2 | tablespoons yeast |

Add all ingredients in Bosch bowl. Add enough flour till dough is clean from sides of bowl. Knead 5 minutes.

Form into 2 loaves. Place in 2 well-oiled bread pans.

Cover and let rise until double. Lower the oven temperature to 350° right before placing in oven.

Bake at 350° for 30-35 minutes.

**Baking Note:** Raisins rehydrated in warm apple juice for 30 minutes prior to adding to this recipe make a more plump and delicious raisin. Drain before adding.

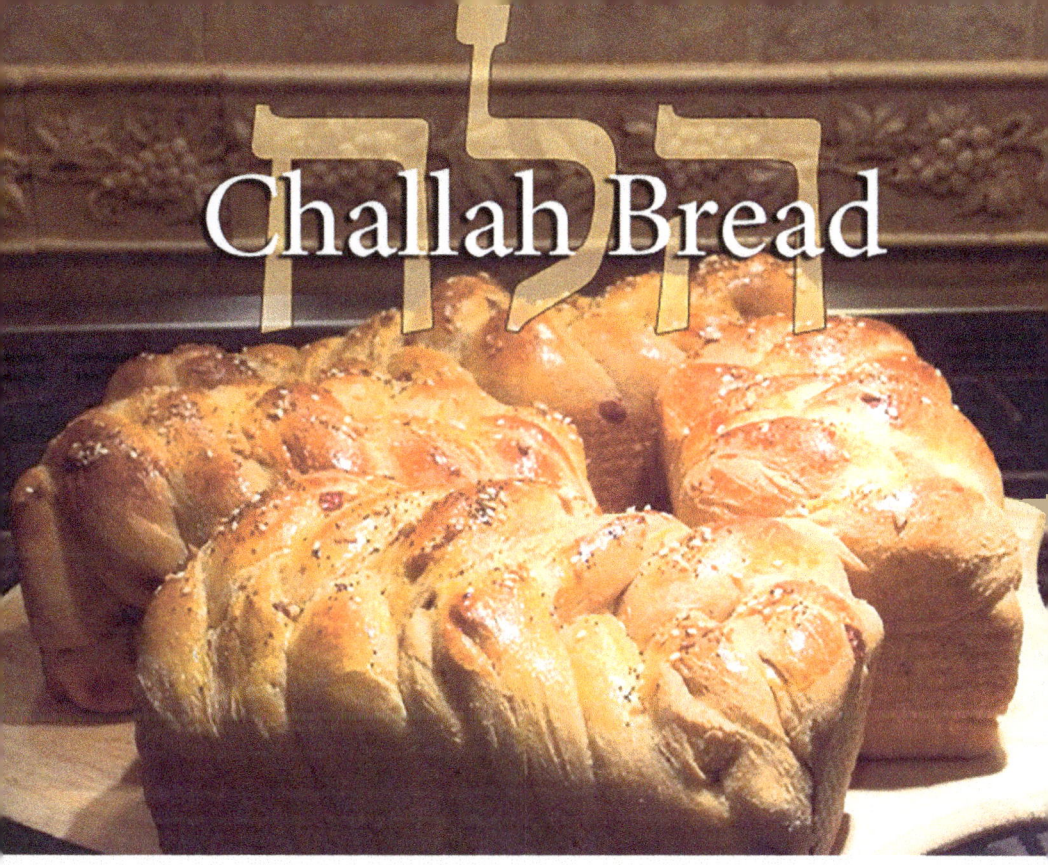

# Challah Bread

## Challah Prayer Bread

On a recent trip to Israel we spent an afternoon making challah bread. This bread making experience was not about mixing and baking: it was about praying.

Each step of the process and each ingredient lent itself to a different prayer. It was heartening and very enriching. It reminded me of my hurried lifestyle as a wife, mother, and entrepreneur. I spend my mornings in prayer but this gave me a chance to expand that prayer. This was a chance to slow down, mix the bread, and pray specifically.

The lessons here are to be cherished, enjoyed and shared with family.

Here is the simple recipe and guidance.

Have ready a bowl for mixing, all ingredients, a towel for your hands and a quiet room.

- The **flour** represents basic provision. It calls us to pray that God will bless us with provision enough to offer assistance to others. We thank him for allowing us to have personal relationship with him – which sustains us. (**1 Kilo**) **7 cups**
- A **handful** of **yeast** represents growth. As it is added it calls us to pray that family members and friends would rise to full potential. We pray against pride and arrogance that puff up.
- A **handful** of **salt** represents discipline. It calls us to pray that anything toxic would be removed from our lives and that we would boldly live for Christ as salt to the nations.
- **Seven spoons** of **sugar** (sucanat) represent a divine amount of all that is sweet and good in our lives. It represents faith and so as it is added we thank God for even the hard times, knowing that if we love him, He can work them for our good.
- After these ingredients are mixed a **handful** of **olive oil**, full and overflowing, is added, poured from the hand little by little, remembering each loved one to the Lord as it is added.
- **Water** binds it all together (**2.5 cups** tepid), representing God's Word. A prayer of submission and surrender is offered as everything is mixed and becomes one whole, bound by His teachings.
- As the dough is **kneaded** pray that stresses would cause family members to wake up to God's reality, growing during times of discipline.
- The dough is divided into three parts representing **mind, body,** and **spirit.** The three are braided together forming a whole. An **egg** is beaten with a bit of water. This wash is painted over the

### Baking with Whole Grain Goodness

loaf, representing renewed life only known through our salvation, covering us completely and forming a shield, as a seal of protection.

Place in prepared pans, let rise and bake at 350°F for 20-30 minutes depending on size. Bake 2 loaves to show double portion of manna.

## 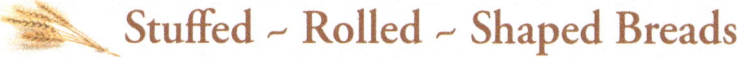 Stuffed ~ Rolled ~ Shaped Breads

Use the Honey Whole Wheat bread dough for these favorite recipes.

Have fun and enjoy!

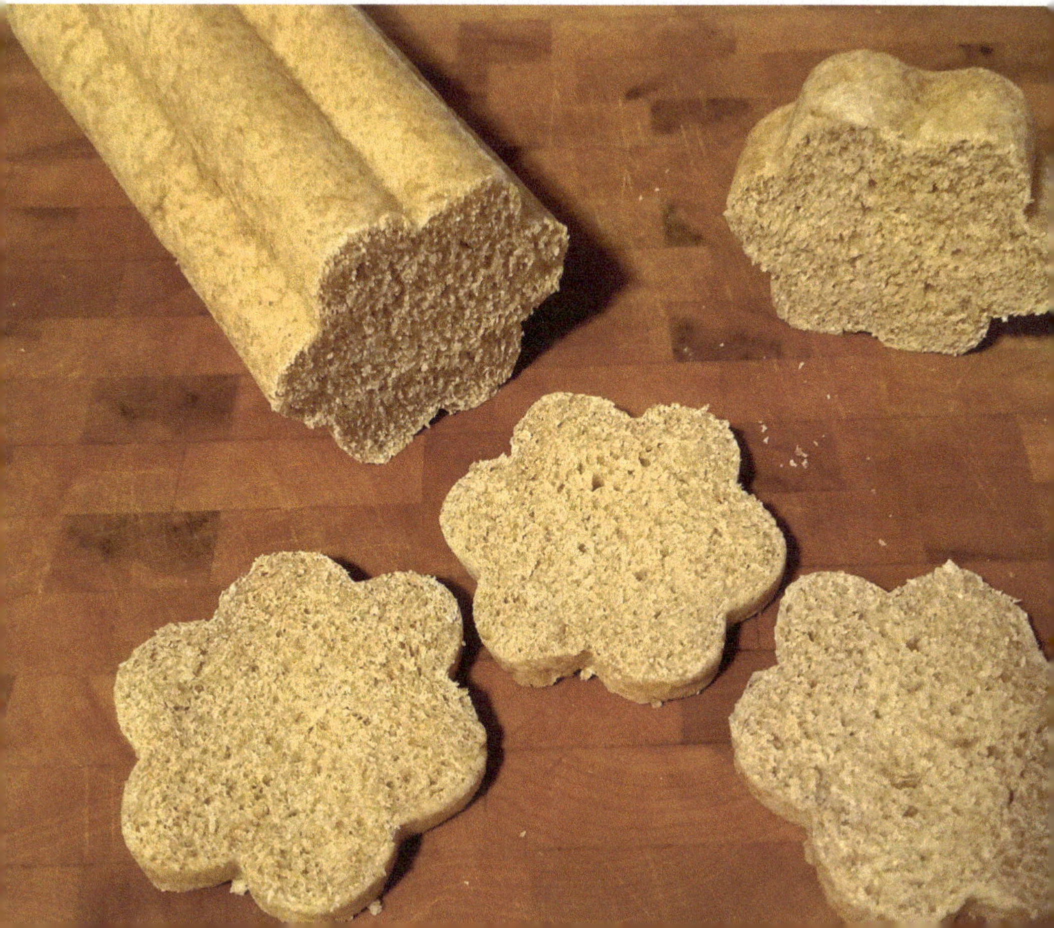

# Hamburger Buns

Cut 1½ pounds bread dough into 8 equal pieces. Form each piece into a ball and place it on a greased or lined baking sheet. Flatten each ball of dough. Brush with a mixture of 1 beaten egg and 1 tablespoon water. Sprinkle with sesame seeds, if desired. Cover lightly and let rise 30 minutes or until doubled. Bake at 350°F for 20-25 minutes or until golden brown.

Any of your favorite bread recipes will make tasty buns. They store well in the freezer for quick lunches. I have tried hot dog buns but it turned out to be too much bread for a single hot dog.

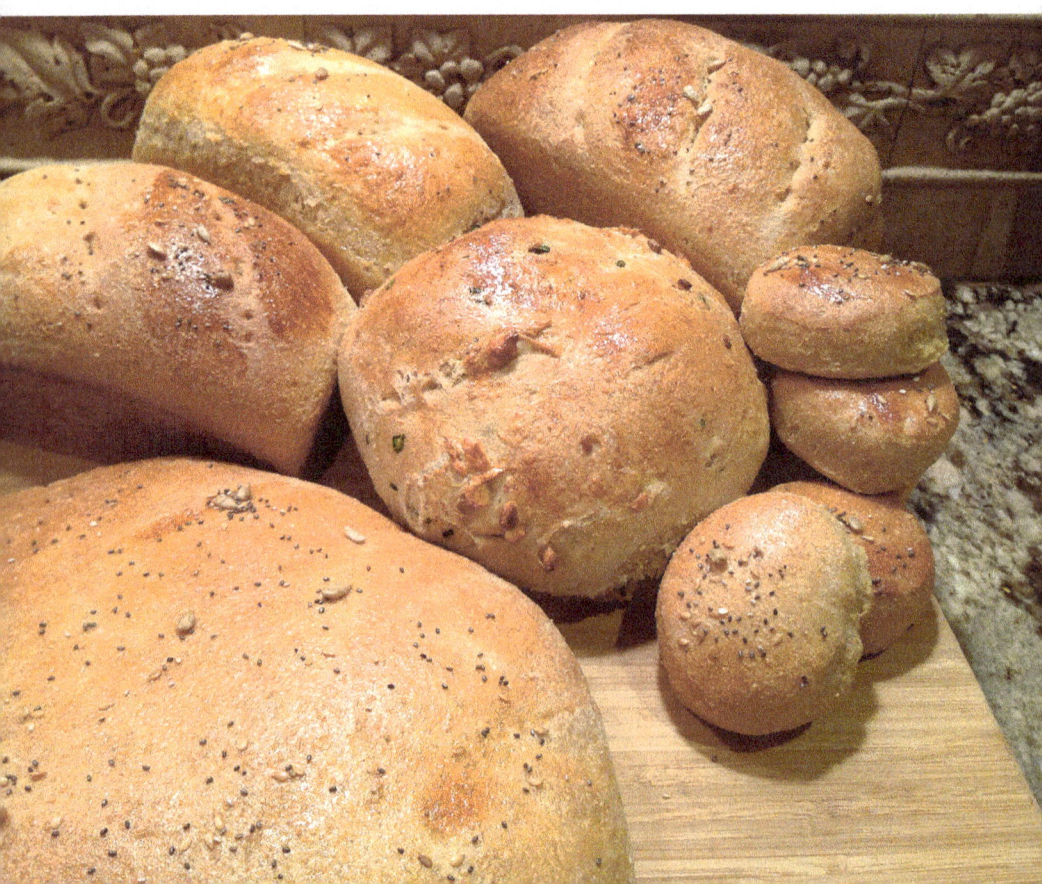

# Family Sandwich

Inspired from cooking friends Phyllis and Shirley and in their book *Healthy Recipes from the Heart of Our Homes*

This is a fun way to feed your friends that is better than a sub sandwich.

The Whole Wheat Honey Bread recipe tastes great in this sandwich.

Use enough dough to roll out into a 12 inch round flat loaf about an inch high. Brush on the following topping.

### *Topping:*
1 egg, beaten and spread over flattened dough
1 tablespoon garlic salt
1 tablespoon dried, minced onion
1 tablespoon sesame seeds

Let rise for 20 minutes.

Bake 425°F for 10-15 minutes.

After the bread cools. Slice the bread horizontally like a huge deli bun and spread with your favorite condiments topped with meat slices, cheese slices, lettuce and tomatoes.

Cut into 12 wedges like a pie.

*Satisfied*

# Feta-Spinach Bread

Inspired from *Healthy Recipes from the Heart of the Home*

Preheat oven to 375°F.

Place in your Bosch mixer, with dough hook:

| | |
|---|---|
| 3 | cups hot water |
| ½ | cup oil |
| ½ | cup honey or maple syrup |
| 1 | tablespoon salt |
| 1 | tablespoon lemon juice |
| 9-10 | cups ground wheat or spelt flour |
| 2 | tablespoons Yeast |

Add flour until dough pulls away from side of the bowl. Knead for 5 minutes.

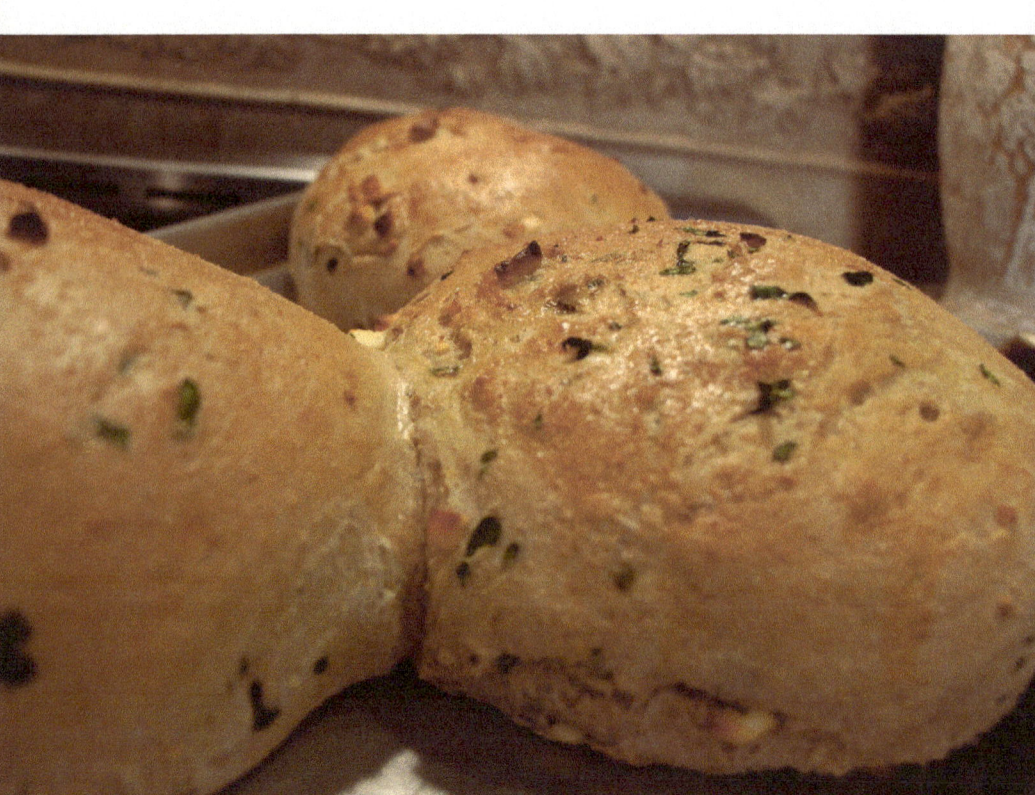

## *Add:*

- 4-6 ounces herb flavored feta cheese
- 10 ounces spinach defrosted (blot spinach with paper towel to remove moisture), or 3 cups finely chopped fresh spinach

Knead lightly only to mix ingredients.

Makes 3 loaves. Let rise for approximately 30 minutes, until it has doubled in size.

Lower heat in oven and bake at 350°F for 30-35 minutes, depending on your oven.

## *Baking Note*

When baking with whole grains increase the amount of herbs and spices in the recipe by up to 50%. White flour is neutral and has no flavor, but whole grain and bean flours can mask the taste of other ingredients.

*Satisfied*

# Cinnamon Bread

Cinnamon
Coconut
Nuts
Chocolate chips

Raisins
Melted butter – 4 ounces
Sucanat – cover all of the dough
Powdered apples

Use a bread recipe from pages 37-42. Roll out dough into a rectangle. Brush the dough with melted butter. Then top with ingredients. All variety of ingredients will taste delicious.

Whole wheat dough has a strong flavor so extra spices are best.

After all ingredients are sprinkled over dough, rollup like a sleeping bag. The cinnamon roll can then be sliced and placed with sides touching for baking or baked as a jelly roll and sliced after it cools.

Bake at 350°F for 30 minutes.

**FRUIT ROLL VARIATION** – blend fresh blueberries (drained), strawberries (drained) and other favorite fruits in a blender or food processor. Add sucanat to preferred taste.

Add ½ teaspoon cinnamon and ¼ cup coconut and mix well.

Add ½ cup nuts – optional.

Spread over rectangle **without** butter and prepare as directed.

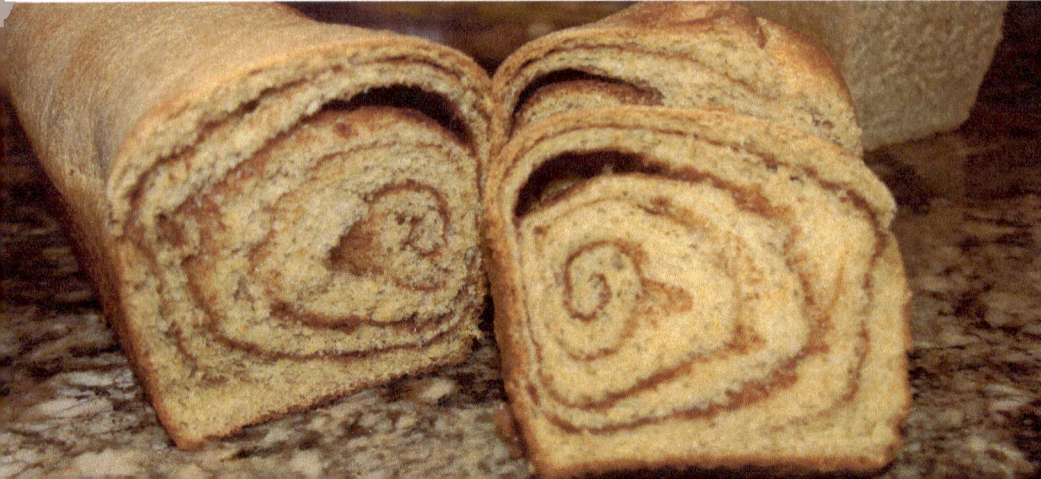

# Garlic Herb Bread

This can be a roll, kneaded in or placed on top
- Garlic seasoning
- Italian seasoning
- Olive oil
- Cheese – any flavor, optional

# Sausage Cheese Bread

- Cooked turkey sausage
- Shredded cheese – farmers is our favorite
- Olive oil or butter
- Italian seasoning

Use a bread recipe from pages 37-42. Roll out dough into a rectangle. Brush a little olive oil or melted butter on the dough. Then add seasonings, cheese and sausage. Roll up like a sleeping bag.

Bake at 350°F for at least 30 minutes or until done.

# Cheese Bread

NOTE: These ingredients are lightly kneaded into the dough. Do not over knead since the dough has already been fully kneaded. Knead only until barely mixed.

- 1 cup shredded cheddar cheese
- Basil, oregano, garlic powder

## Baking Note

After milling grains and legumes, refrigerate or freeze any leftover flour to preserve as many nutrients as possible. Flour may be stored up to 2 weeks in the refrigerator or 3-6 months in the freezer.

*Satisfied*

# Braided Apple Cinnamon

Chopped apples
Cinnamon
Sucanat
Nuts

Directions for braid:

Use a bread recipe from pages 37-42.

Divide dough into thirds

Roll out each third and put cinnamon and chopped apples on it.

Roll up like a sleeping bag, And then braid the three together.

Bake at 350°F for at least 20–25 minutes.

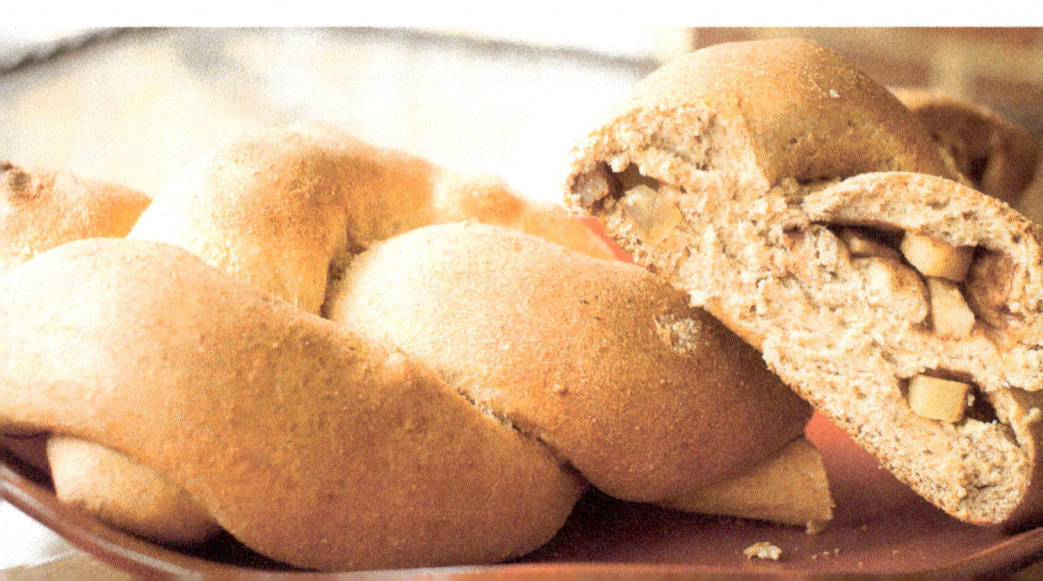

# Spinach-Cheese French Bread

| | |
|---|---|
| 1 | small onion, chopped |
| 2 | tablespoons butter |
| 1 | package 10 oz. frozen chopped spinach, thawed and squeezed dry – or fresh spinach cooked and chopped |
| 1 | cup mozzarella cheese, shredded – Farmers cheese will work well |
| 1 | cup shredded cheddar cheese |
| 1 | cup chopped fresh mushrooms |
| ⅛ | teaspoon salt |
| ⅛ | teaspoon pepper |
| ⅛ | teaspoon hot pepper sauce – optional |
| 1 | loaf French bread halved lengthwise |
| ½ | cup parmesan cheese |

In a large skillet, sauté onion in butter until tender. Remove from heat. Stir in spinach, cheeses, mushrooms, salt, pepper and hot pepper sauce. Spoon onto bread halves.

Place on an ungreased baking sheet. Sprinkle with Parmesan Cheese. Bake 350°F for 10-15 minutes or until cheese is melted.

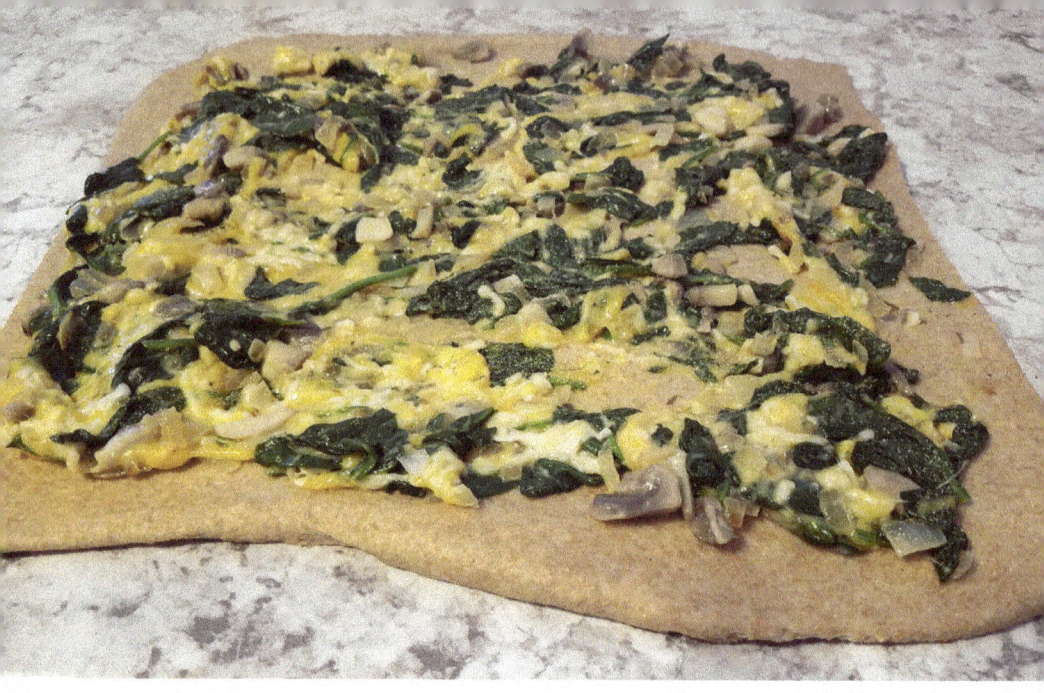

## Spinach Cheese Stromboli

Use a bread recipe from pages 37-42. Follow step 1 on page 53 for sautéing onions and adding spinach, cheese, mushrooms and seasonings. Roll out dough into a rectangle and spoon the spinach cheese mixture to cover 2/3 of the dough. Then the dough can be rolled up like a sleeping bag or the edges can be rolled and made into an edge and baked like a pizza.

Bake at 350°F for 15 minutes.

## Stuffed Reuben Bread

- ⅓ cup Thousand Island Salad Dressing
- 1 cup sauerkraut, drained
- ½ pound Swiss cheese
- ⅓ pound corned beef

Follow Stromboli directions.

## Turkey Stromboli

1-2 tablespoons Dijon mustard
2   cups Swiss cheese
½   pound smoked turkey slices

Follow Stromboli directions.

## Ranch Pizza Pinwheels

Pizza crust dough- you can use the recipe in the Healthy Treasures cookbook

- ¼ cup prepared ranch salad dressing – make your own for better flavor and health
- ½ cup shredded Colby Monterey jack cheese – or cheese of your choice
- ½ cup diced or sliced meat – your choice – pizza type
- ¼ cup chopped green onions

*Dressings are best made from real ingredients. See recipes for Thousand Island and Ranch in the Healthy Treasures Cookbook*

On a lightly floured surface, roll pizza dough into a 12 inch x 10 inch rectangle. Spread ranch dressing evenly to within ¼ of edges. Sprinkle with cheese, meat, and onions. Roll up jelly-roll style, starting with long side.

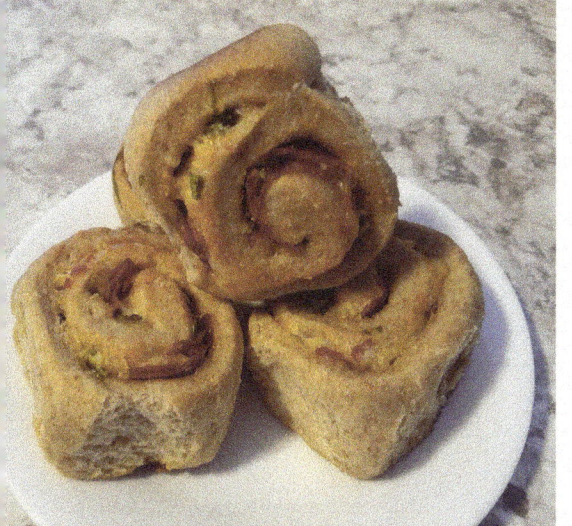

Cut into 1 inch slices. Place cut side down on a greased baking sheet.

Bake at 425°F for 10-13 minutes or until lightly browned.

Serve warm with pizza sauce or additional ranch dressing if desired.

Refrigerate leftovers.

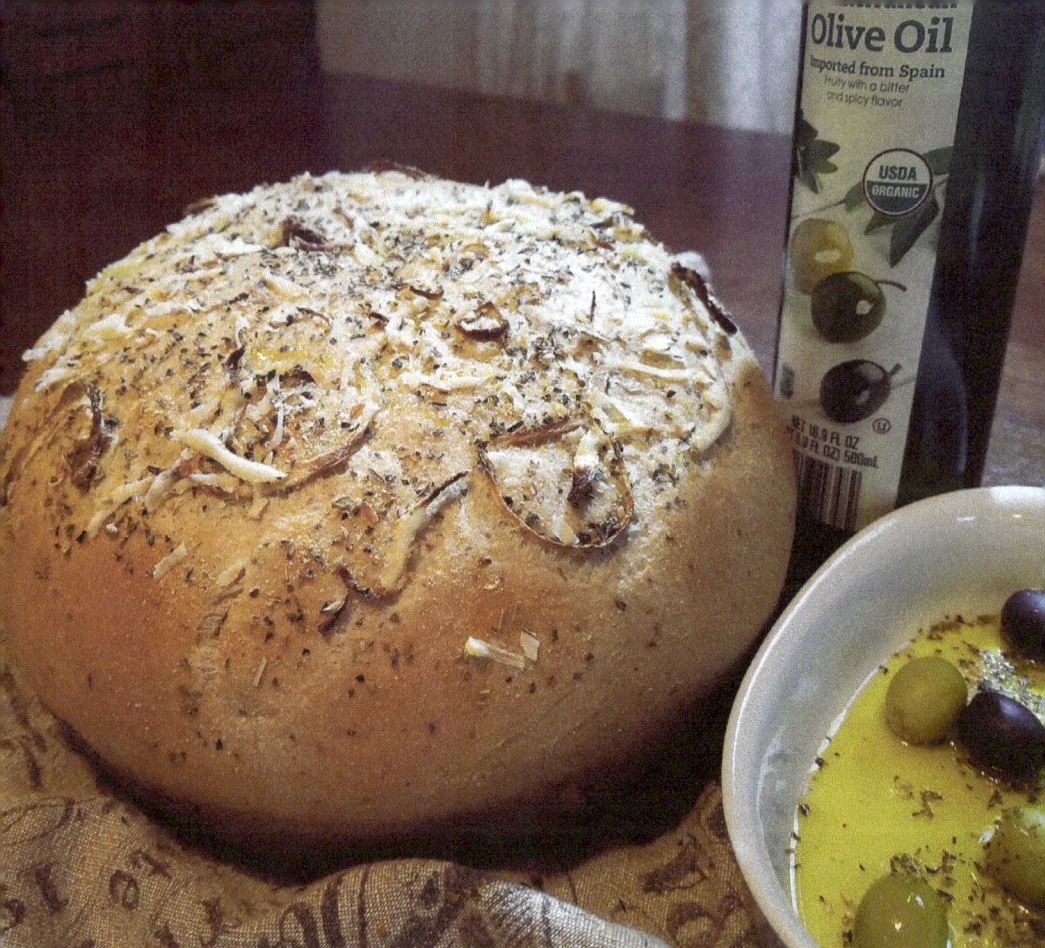

## Italian Bread

Make bread following any of the recipes in this book.

Place the dough on a round cheese cake pan or plain round cake pan.

As it rises, add Italian seasoning, a bit of garlic powder plus thinly sliced onions on top. Red onions make it look very fancy, like Panera's Focaccia bread. Cheese could be added also.

A Christmas bread could also have red and green peppers on top.

Cook as directed for bread.

# Garlic Knots

Prepare your favorite bread dough. Use fresh herbs finely chopped for a flavorful delight.

| | |
|---|---|
| 8 | cloves garlic – minced |
| ¼ | cup olive oil |
| ¼ | cup basil |
| ⅛ | cup rosemary |
| ⅛ | cup fresh oregano |
| ½ | teaspoons salt |
| ½ | cup - fresh grated parmesan cheese |

When dough is ready (kneaded), place approximately 1 tablespoon sized pieces on baking sheet. Bake in 350°F oven for about 10 minutes – before browned.

In a large bowl pour in olive oil, add raw chopped herbs, salt, and cheese. Stir with whisk. Toss in the baked dough balls to fully coat. Serve warm.

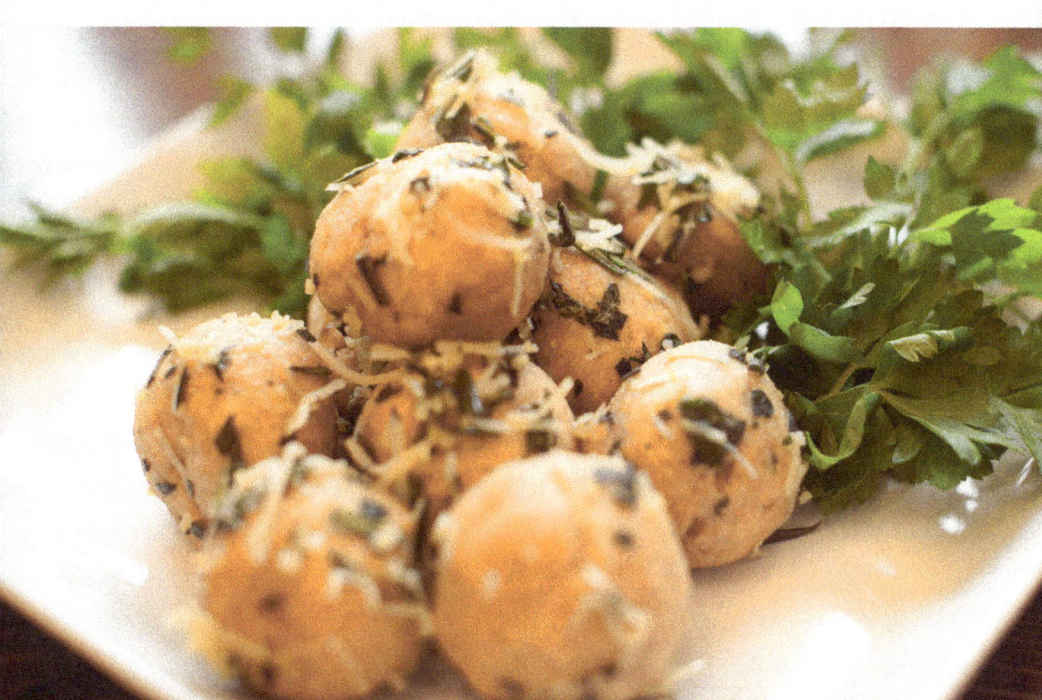

## Cinnamon Croutons

The perfect change from the usual garlic croutons.

>   Day old bread - sliced
>   Melted butter
>   Cinnamon / sucanat mixture

Spread melted butter on both sides of bread slices. Cut into small cubes. Place cubes in plastic bag and add cinnamon/ Sucanat mixture. Shake to coat all cubes.

Place on baking sheet in a single layer.

Bake at 375°F for 10 minutes.

## Garlic Croutons

Perfect use for stale bread!

| | |
|---|---|
| 3 | cups day old bread |
| ¼ | cup olive oil |
| 3 | tablespoons grated parmesan cheese |
| ¼ | teaspoon garlic powder |
| ¼ | teaspoon salt |
| | Black pepper to taste |

Preheat the oven to 375º F.

In a large bowl, combine the bread, olive oil, parmesan cheese, garlic powder, salt, and pepper. Toss well to distribute the ingredients.

Spread the bread cubes out on a sheet pan, giving them plenty of space in between. Bake the bread cubes for about 10 minutes, or until slightly golden brown and crisp. Keep in mind that older bread will brown quicker, so color is a good indication of when it's done.

Remove the croutons from the oven and enjoy! Perfect topping for soups and salads. Sometimes they are good to just pop in your mouth.

## Baking Note

Bean flours provide extra protein and may be added in small quantities to any baked goods. You can replace up to 10% - 25% of the wheat flour in your recipes with almost any bean, pea, or lentil flour.

Croutons made from Russian Black Rye Bread.

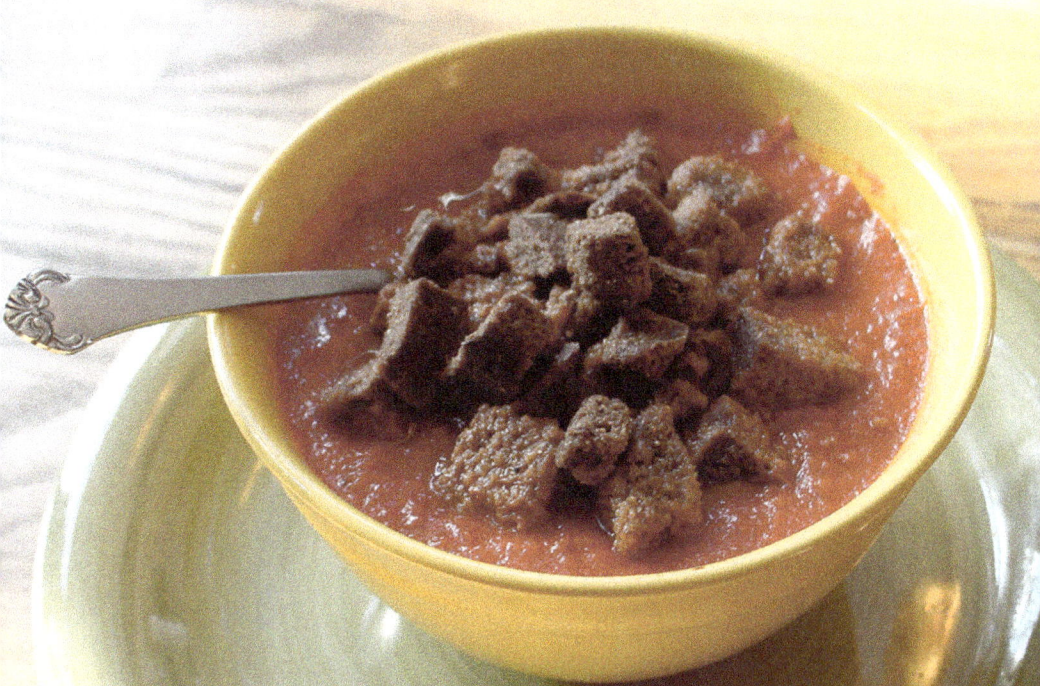

## Better Butters

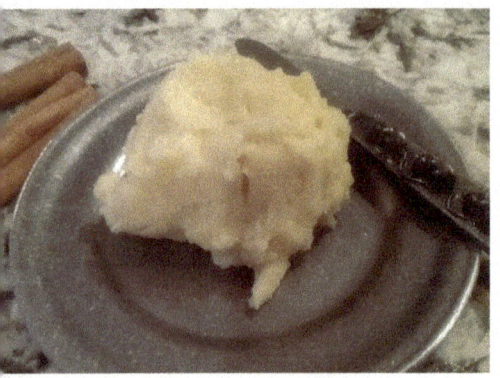

### Cinnamon Butter

8 ounces soft butter

1 cup honey

¼ teaspoon cinnamon

Combine in blender until smooth. Store in refrigerator.

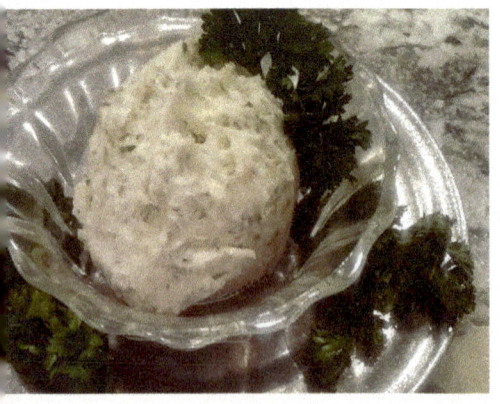

### Herbed Butter

8 ounces soft butter

2 teaspoons fresh parsley, chopped

2 teaspoons fresh oregano, chopped

1 teaspoon fresh basil, chopped

1 garlic clove, minced

Combine in blender until smooth. Store in refrigerator.

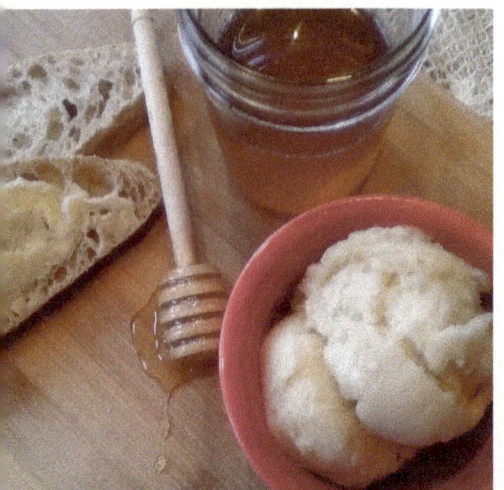

### Honey Butter

8 ounces soft butter

1 cup honey – less is ok

Combine in blender until smooth.

Store in refrigerator

## Lemon Butter

| | |
|---|---|
| 8 | ounces soft butter |
| ½ | teaspoon fresh thyme, finely chopped |
| 1 | teaspoon lemon zest |
| ½ | small lemon squeezed (more if desired) |

Combine in blender until smooth.

Store in refrigerator.

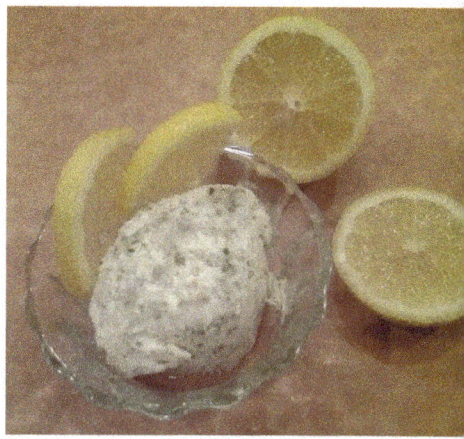

## Pecan Butter

| | |
|---|---|
| 8 | ounces soft butter |
| 4 | tablespoons toasted pecans, finely chopped |
| 2 | tablespoon sucanat |

Combine in blender until smooth.

Store in refrigerator.

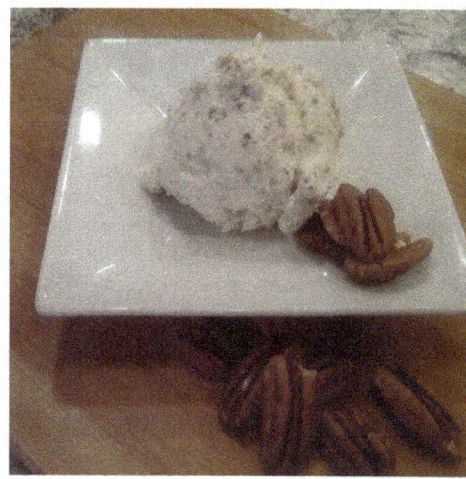

## Strawberry Butter

| | |
|---|---|
| 1 | cup strawberries – thawed, drained |
| ¼ | cup honey |
| 8 | ounces soft butter |

Combine in blender until smooth. Store in refrigerator.

Other variations could be blueberries, raspberries, cranberries or peaches.

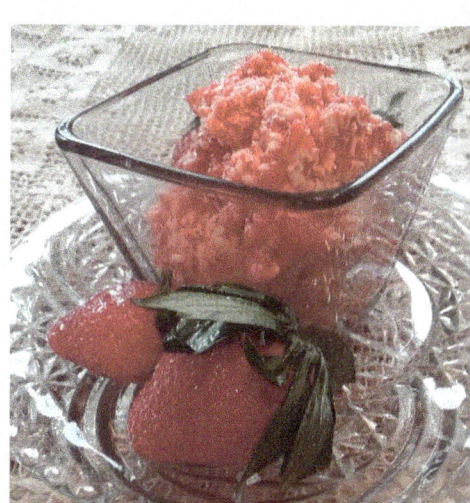

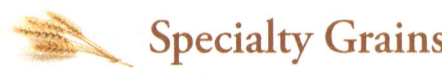

## 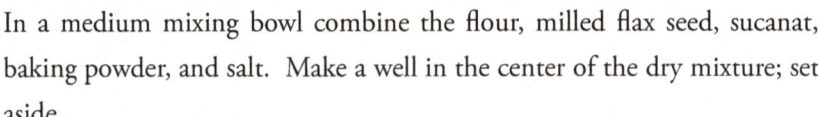 Specialty Grains

# Easy Nutritious Pancakes GF

*Your kids are sure to love!*

Prep: 10 minutes ~ Makes 8-10 pancakes

- 1 cup freshly milled buckwheat flour
- 1-2 tablespoon milled flax seed
- 1 tablespoon sucanat
- 2 teaspoon baking powder
- ¼ teaspoon salt
- 1 beaten egg
- 1 cup milk
- 2 tablespoons olive oil
- ½ cup purée of choice: sweet potato, pumpkin, or banana

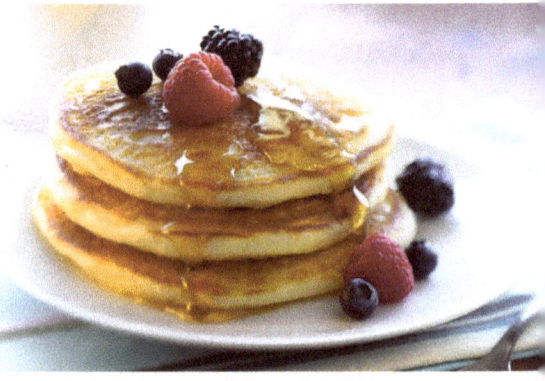

In a medium mixing bowl combine the flour, milled flax seed, sucanat, baking powder, and salt. Make a well in the center of the dry mixture; set aside.

In another medium mixing bowl combine the egg, milk, and oil. Add egg mixture all at once to the dry mixture. Stir just until moistened (batter should be lumpy).

Mix in Purée of choice.

Pour about ¼ cup of batter onto a hot, lightly greased griddle or heavy skillet. Cook! Pancakes are ready to turn when the tops are bubbly and they are slightly "set" or the edges are slightly dry. *With an added purée they will take a bit longer to cook due to the added moisture.

# Family Table Talk

*And they were continually devoting themselves
to fellowship and to breaking bread.*

Topics for discussion starters at the family table.

Where is one place you would like to visit?

What Bible stories can you share about bread?

Read an ongoing story.

What is your favorite phrase to hear or say?

What worries you most?

How can we help our neighbors?

What is the funniest thing that happened to you today?

How did you see God at work today?

What happened to you today that you enjoyed?

Make a list of fun activities the family can do if they save money by turning out lights and turning off electrical items.

Share ways to help more people outside the family: kids, families, pastor, mailman, etc.

Share ways to be more helpful around the home.

In the winter share ideas for planting a garden and what plants you would like to see grow and taste.

Discuss a current events story and share how God might be working in it.

If you had $1,000 what would you do with the money?

Name one physical feature about yourself that you like.

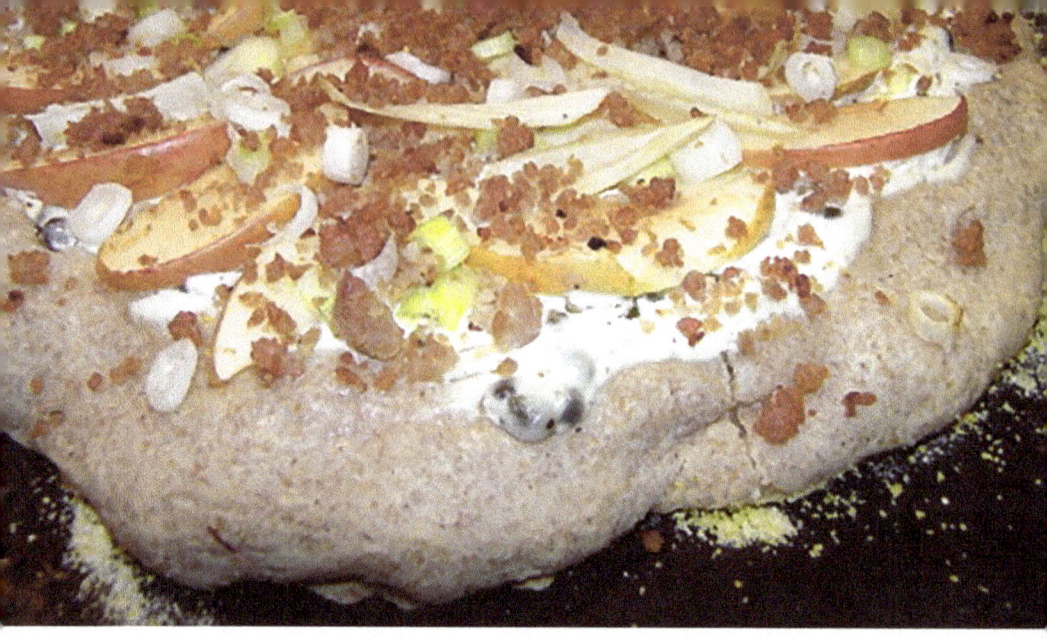

# Spelt Crust Pizza

Inspired from *Epicurious* website.

## Ingredients:

- 2 cups whole grain spelt flour (8 oz.) or other grains such as kamut, wheat, rye.
- 2 teaspoons baking powder
- ¾ teaspoon fine sea salt
- ½ teaspoon sucanat
- ½ cup cream cheese
- ½ cup sour cream
- ¼ cup whole milk
- 2 tablespoons extra-virgin olive oil
- 1 large egg
- Coarse cornmeal, if using a pizza peel
- ¾ teaspoons freshly ground black pepper
- 1 Granny Smith apple, halved, cored, and sliced very thinly
- 1 fennel bulb, halved lengthwise, cored, and sliced very thinly
- 4 ounces seasoned turkey sausage, cooked and crumbled
- Extra-virgin olive oil, for brushing

# Directions:

First, make the dough.

**TO PREPARE THE DOUGH BY HAND.** Whisk together the spelt flour, baking powder, salt, and sucanat in a large bowl. Make a well in the center. In a small bowl, combine the cream cheese and sour cream, milk, olive oil, and the egg and beat with a fork until smooth.

Pour the cream cheese and sour cream mixture into the well. Combine with a fork, stirring from the center and gradually incorporating the flour from the sides until a moist dough comes together.

**TO PREPARE THE DOUGH IN the BOSCH:** In the Bosch cream the cream cheese, sour cream, milk, oil and egg till smooth. Add dry ingredients. Mix till ball forms – if not forming in 1 minute add a little more flour. The dough will be fairly moist. Knead for 2 minutes in the Bosch to get smooth yet tacky dough. Allow dough to rest for 30 – 45 minutes to allow the bran to soften. (If in a hurry you can bypass this step).

Place a baking stone on a rack on the bottom shelf and preheat oven to 425 °F. Liberally sprinkle pizza peel with coarse cornmeal. Finely chop the white and light green parts of the green onions until you have ½ cup. Combine them with the sour cream, capers and ¼ teaspoon of the pepper in a small bowl. Finely chop the dark green parts as well for garnish.

Knead dough in Bosch for another 1 to 2 minutes till smooth.

Using a rolling pin, roll the dough into an elongated pizza, 11 x 8 inches about ¼ inches thick. Do this gradually, occasionally turning the dough over and rolling it out further, lightly flouring your work surface and the rolling pin each time. Place the dough on the pizza peel. Spread half of the sour cream

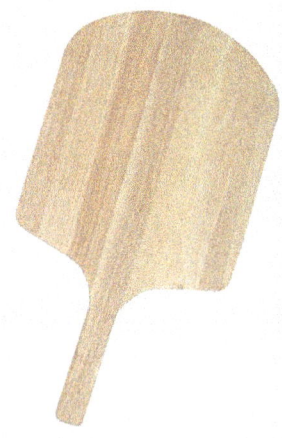

topping across, leaving a ½ inch border. Cover with half of the apple slices, top with half of the fennel slices and sprinkle with half of the sausage. Brush border with oil.

Slide the dough onto the baking stone and bake until the fennel just starts to brown at the edges and the rim turns golden brown and starts to crisp (it should yield when pressed with a finger) about 15 minutes. Use a large spatula to lift the edges of the pizza so you can slide the peel underneath; carefully transfer the pizza to a wooden board. Sprinkle with half of the reserved green onions and the pepper. Cut with a sharp knife and serve at once. Repeat with the second pizza.

## Toppings

4 or 5 green onions
1    cup sour cream
¼    cup drained nonpareil capers

# Cornbread

¾    cup freshly milled flour
¾    cup freshly milled corn meal
¾    teaspoon salt
2½   teaspoons baking powder
¾    cup milk
2    tablespoons honey
1    egg
2-3  tablespoons melted butter

Combine dry ingredients. Add milk, honey, egg and melted butter. Mix well. Bake in a 10 inch greased pan in a preheated oven at 425°F for 25 minutes.

# Ezekiel Grains

Inspired from BreadBeckers.com

| | |
|---|---|
| 2½ | cups hard red wheat |
| 1½ | cups spelt or rye (Biblically, spelt was used, Ezekiel 4:9) |
| ½ | cup barley (hulled barley) |
| ¼ | cup millet |
| ¼ | cup lentils (green preferred) |
| 2 | tablespoons great northern beans |
| 2 | tablespoons red kidney beans |
| 2 | tablespoons pinto beans |

Stir the above ingredients very well. Grind all in your favorite Nutrimill.

| | | | |
|---|---|---|---|
| 4 | cups lukewarm water | 1 | cup honey |
| ½ | cup oil | 2 | teaspoons salt |
| | freshly milled flour from above mixture of grains | | |
| 2 | tablespoons yeast | | |

In large bowl, combine water, honey, oil and salt. Add all of the flour and yeast. Stir or knead until well kneaded about 10 minutes. This is a batter type bread and will not form a smooth ball.

Pour into greased pans. You may use 2 large loaf pans or 3 medium loaf pans or 2 9 x 13 pans. Let rise in a warm place for one hour or until the dough is about ¼ inch from the top of the pan. Do not over rise! If it rises too much it will overflow the pan while baking. Bake at 350°F for 45-50 minutes for loaf pans and 35-40 for brownie pans.

Fruits, nuts, and cinnamon can be added to this recipe.

## Baking Note

Grains may be mixed and milled together at the same time. Choose grains of similar size for best results. Try a variety of flour mixtures to add variety, flavor and texture to your recipes.

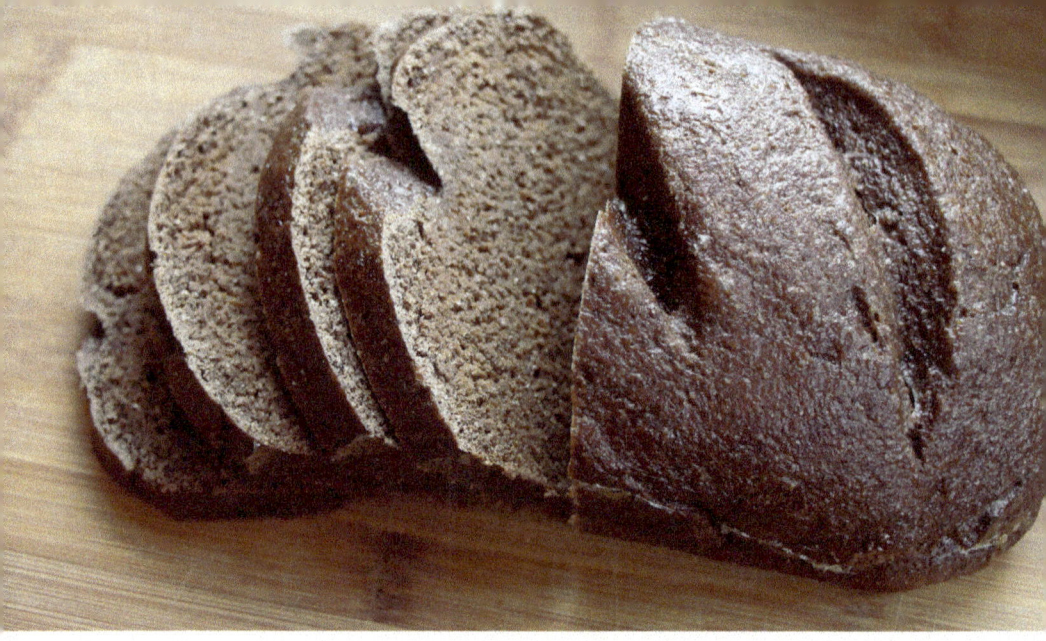

# Russian Black Rye Bread

Recipe inspired from *Homemade Matters*,

1 ¼ cups warm water

2 tablespoons apple cider vinegar

¼ cup molasses

¼ cup honey

2 tablespoons cocoa powder

¼ cup butter, melted

2 teaspoons salt

1 tablespoons dried onion flakes

1 tablespoons caraway seeds, crushed

¼ teaspoons fennel seeds, crushed

1 tablespoons yeast

2 cups rye flour

2-3 cups whole wheat flour

Cornmeal for sprinkling pan

## Glaze

½ cup cold water

1 teaspoon cornstarch (non-GMO)

In Bosch mixing bowl fitted with dough hook mix all ingredients except wheat flour. Gradually add wheat flour, mixing on speed 2 until the dough pulls away from the sides of the bowl.

Knead for 6-8 minutes.

Remove dough and place on an oiled surface. Shape into loaf and place on a greased baking sheet sprinkled with cornmeal. With a knife, cut slits in the loaf and cover loosely with plastic wrap. Let rise until doubled. Bake at 350°F for 40 – 50 minutes until the internal temperature reaches 180 185 °F.

While bread is baking, combine water and corn starch in a small saucepan and cook until thickened. Remove baked bread from the oven, quickly brush with cornstarch glaze and return it to the oven for 2-3 minutes. This will set the glaze and create a chewier crust. Remove from oven to a cooling rack.

## Baking Note

Offset strong-tasting flours (quinoa, millet, rice, beans) by mixing them with mild flour (hard, soft wheat, oat kamut, spelt).

*Satisfied*

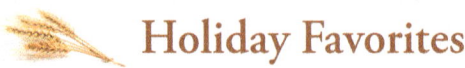 Holiday Favorites

# Almond Raspberry Cheese Bread

Recipe from *Wildflour* by Denise Fidler

| | |
|---|---|
| 3 | cups freshly milled hard white wheat flour |
| 2 | cups freshly milled soft white pastry flour |
| ½ | cup honey |
| 1 | tablespoons yeast |
| ½ | teaspoon salt |
| ½ | cup butter, cut into small pieces |
| ⅓ | cup milk |
| ¼ | cup water |
| 3 | eggs |
| 1½ | cups sliced and toasted almonds |
| 1 | cup raspberry jam or your favorite |

# Cream Cheese Filling

| | |
|---|---|
| 2 – 8 | ounce packages cream cheese, softened |
| ½ | cup sucanat with honey |
| ⅛ | cup flour |
| 1 | eggs whites |
| 1 | teaspoon grated lemon peel |

Beat until smooth.

In heavy-duty mixer bowl with dough hook attachment or large bowl if kneading by hand combine 2 cups flour, honey, yeast, and salt. Heat butter, milk and water until 120° -130°. Butter does not need to melt all the way. Add to mixer bowl. Stir in eggs, 2 cups of the almonds and enough additional flour to make a smooth dough and knead 5-7 minutes in mixer bowl or 12-15 minutes by hand until dough is smooth and satiny.

Divide dough into 2 equal pieces and roll out into rectangles. Spread cream cheese filling down the center third of each rectangle and spread raspberry jam on top. Along each side cut one inch strips from edge of filling to edge of dough.

Starting at one end, alternately fold strips from each side across filling toward opposite end. Transfer to greased sheets and cover and let rise until double and bake at 375° for about 25 minutes.

Drizzle with powdered sugar glaze and toasted sliced almonds.

## Glaze

Combine in bowl:

| | |
|---|---|
| 1 | cups powdered sugar (honey crystals can be placed in a blender to become a powder) |
| ¼ | cup milk |
| ½ | teaspoon vanilla |

Beat until smooth.

## Baking Note

Whole grain flours absorb liquid more slowly than white flour. If your pancake batter appears runny, wait 5 minutes. The batter will thicken as it sits. Adding too much flour too soon will make the batter dry.

## Apple Pie French Toast

This will quickly become your new Christmas morning favorite.

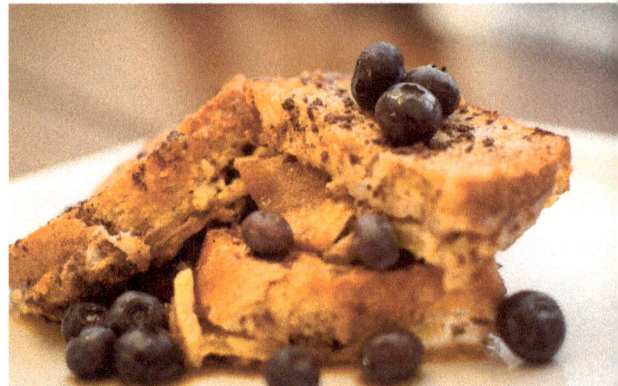

- 1 stick butter
- 1 cup (240 ml) sucanat with honey or honey crystals
- 6 slices whole wheat bread
- 6 eggs
- 1¼ cups (300 ml) milk
- 1 teaspoon vanilla
- 1 teaspoon salt
- 1 tablespoon cinnamon
- 6 apples, peeled and thinly sliced

Melt butter in 13" x 9" pan.

Add sucanat to butter and spread over pan.

Place apple slices on top of butter mixture in a double layer.

Place bread slices on top of apples.

In mixing bowl, beat eggs.

Add milk, vanilla, salt, and cinnamon. Pour egg mixture over bread slices. Refrigerate overnight.

In the morning, preheat oven to 350°F

Bake uncovered for 35-40 minutes.

Makes 8 servings

# Cranberry Quinoa Scones

- 1 cup quinoa flour (grind fresh in Mock Mill)
- 1 cup spelt flour
- ⅓ cup maple syrup
- ½ teaspoon salt
- ½ teaspoon baking soda
- 1½ teaspoon baking powder
- ½ cup butter – softened
- ½ cup buttermilk, plus extra for tops
- 2 teaspoons orange zest for top of scones
- ½ cup cranberries

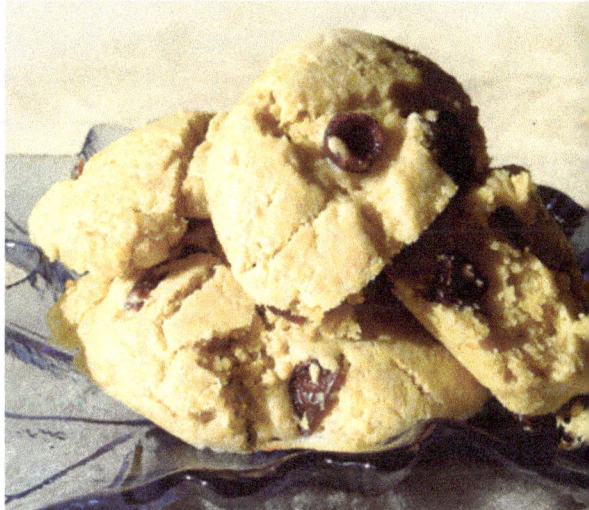

## Instructions

In Bosch mixer with cookie paddles, mix above ingredients until moistened.

Place dough on lightly floured board and roll to ¾" thick.

Using a 2" round cookie cutter, cut out circles of dough.

Place on parchment paper.

Brush tops with buttermilk.

Preheat oven then bake at 425°F for 12-15 minutes or until golden brown.

# Cranberry Wreaths

Recipe from *Wildflour* by Denise Fidler

These are an attractive addition to your holiday goodies!

One Whole Wheat Honey Recipe using equal amounts of spelt and kamut.

Roll dough into two 21 inch by 12 inch rectangles. Spread cranberry filling over dough to within ½ inch of the edges. Fold length-wise in thirds to enclose the filling making a 12 x 7 inch rectangle. Press edges together to seal.

Cut dough into twelve 1 inch strips. Holding ends of strips, twist three times. Pinch together ends of each twisted strip to form wreaths; place on greased baking sheets. Cover; let rise in warm place until almost doubled about 45 minutes. Bake at 400°F for 12-15 minutes or until done. Cook and drizzle with glaze.

# Cranberry Filling

In sauce pan combine

- 2 cups finely chopped cranberries
- 1 cup sucanat with honey or sugar
- 4 teaspoon freshly grated orange peel

Bring to boil and then simmer over low heat until very thick being sure to stir frequently. Let cool.

# Glaze

- 2 cups powdered sucanat or sugar
- ½ cup milk
- 1 teaspoon vanilla

# Cream Cheese Pumpkin Muffins

Recipe from *Wildflour* by Denise Fidler

Here is a special holiday treat delicately rich and delicious.

## Filling

| | |
|---|---|
| 5 | ounces cream cheese, softened, |
| 1 | small egg |
| 2 | tablespoons sucanat with honey |

Blend ingredients till smooth and creamy. Set aside.

## Topping

| | |
|---|---|
| ⅓ | cup dried coconut, unsweetened |
| ¼ | cup chopped pecans |
| 1½ | tablespoon Sucanat |

Mix ingredients and set aside.

In mixing bowl combine these dry ingredients:

| | |
|---|---|
| 1½ | cups soft whole wheat pastry flour or hard white whole wheat flour |
| ½ | cup sucanat with honey or sugar |
| 1 | teaspoon baking powder |
| 1 | teaspoon cinnamon |
| ¼ | teaspoon salt |
| ⅛ | teaspoon baking soda |

Mix the liquid ingredients together in separate bowl:

| | |
|---|---|
| 1 | egg |
| ¾ | cup pumpkin puree |
| 2 | tablespoon oil |
| ½ | teaspoon vanilla |

# Satisfied

Fold the liquid ingredients into the dry flour mixture.

Fill muffin pans one third full with batter and make an indention in center of each muffin. Place a spoonful of cream cheese filling into the indention. Cover with remaining muffin mixture.

Sprinkle topping over each and bake at 400°F for about 18-20 minutes.

Makes 9-10 muffins.

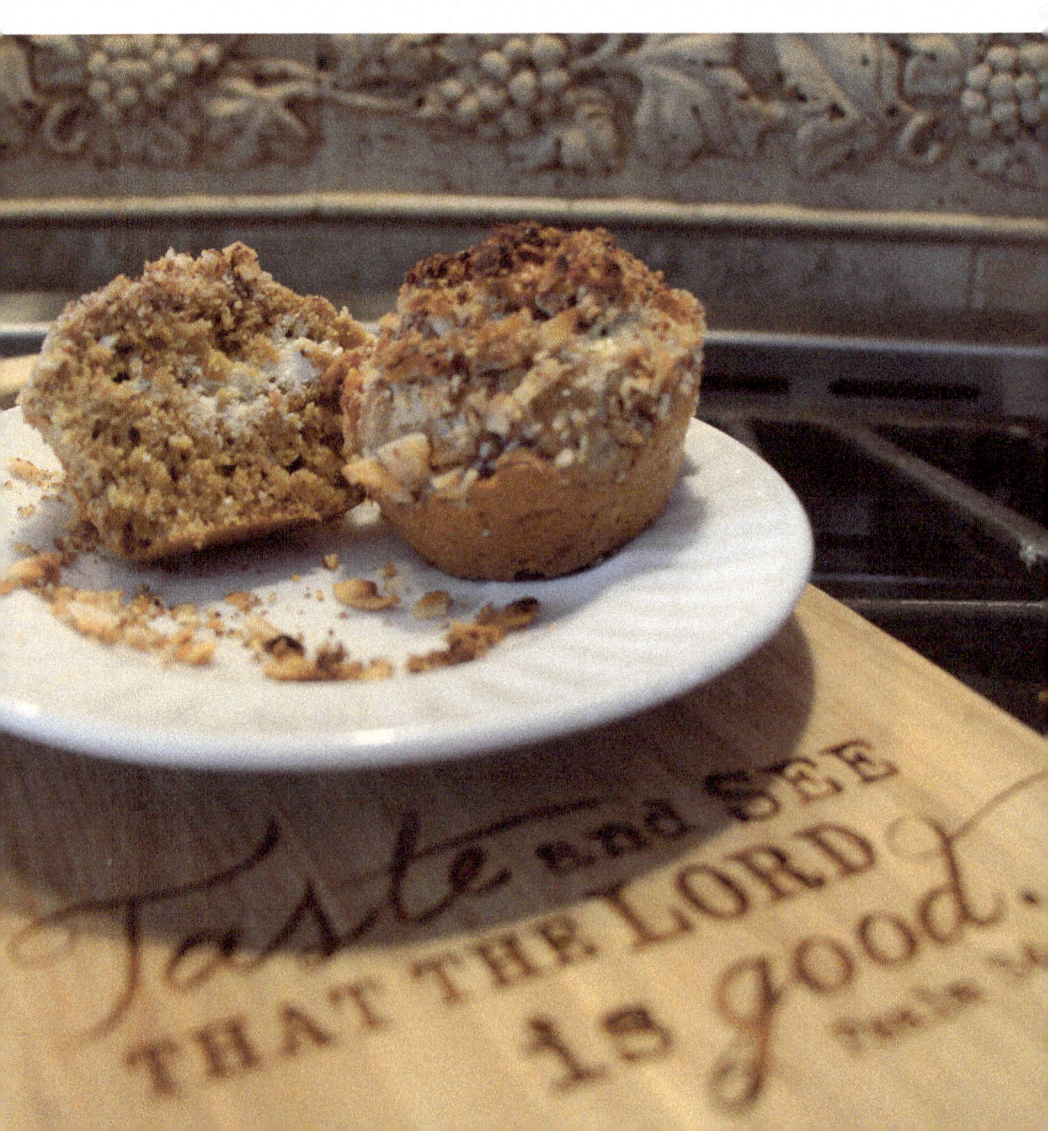

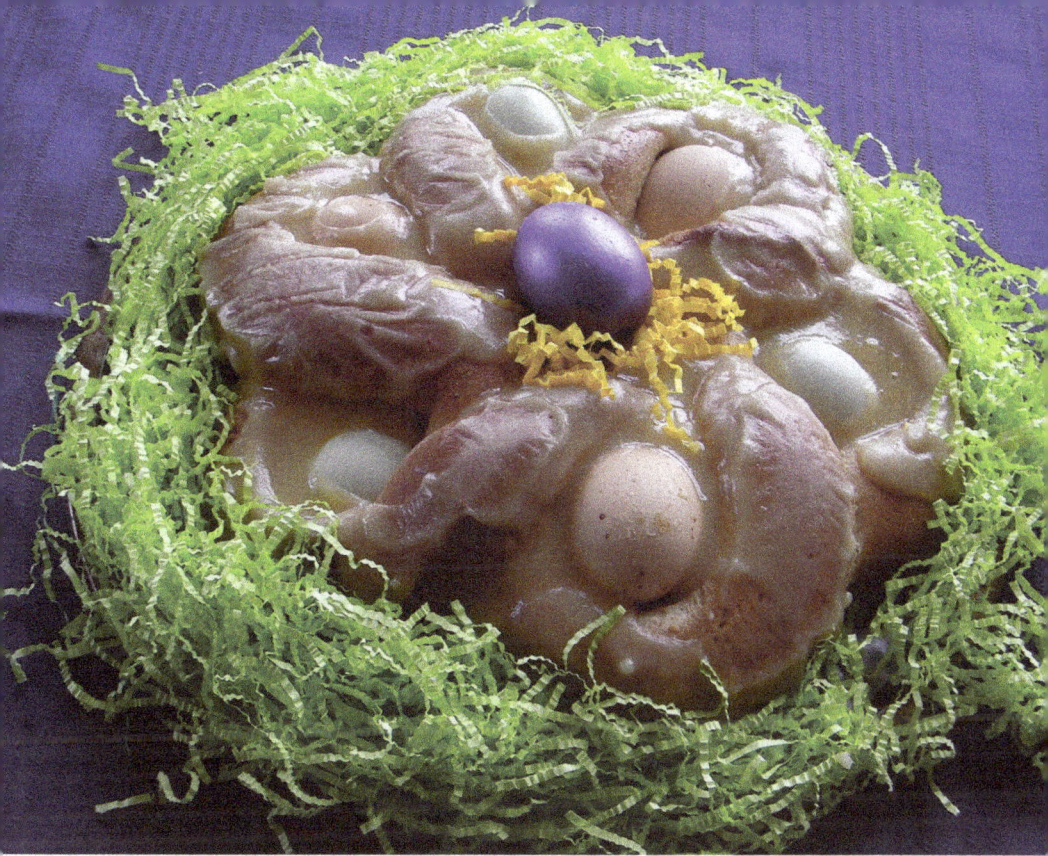

# Easter Egg Nest Bread

Recipe from *Wildflour* by Denise Fidler

Such a fun recipe – the eggs cook as the bread bakes!

| | |
|---|---|
| 1½ | cups water |
| ⅔ | cup milk |
| ½ | cup butter |

Heat these liquids to 120°-125°F and set aside.

| | |
|---|---|
| 5 | cups freshly milled hard white wheat flour |
| 5 | cups freshly milled soft pastry flour |
| ⅔ | cup honey |
| 2 | tablespoons yeast |
| 2 | tablespoons freshly grated orange peel |
| 1 | tablespoons orange oil |

| | |
|---|---|
| 2 | tablespoons salt |
| 18 | eggs |
| 1 | cup chopped toasted almonds |
| 2 | tablespoons Water |
| | Orange icing – recipe follows |

In heavy-duty mixer bowl (Bosch) with dough hook attachment or large mixing bowl if kneading by hand, combine heated mixture, 3 cups flour, honey, yeast, orange peel, orange oil and salt. Stir in 2 eggs, almonds, and enough remaining flour to make a soft dough. Knead 5-7 minutes in mixer or 12-15 minutes by hand. Cover and rest 10 minutes.

Divide dough into 4 pieces. Roll each into a 30 inch rope. Loosely twist two ropes together. Place ropes on large greased sheet. Shape into circles and pinch ends together to seal.

Place 7 clean eggs evenly spaced on each circle of dough pressing between ropes in twist. Cover and let rise until double.

Beat remaining eggs with 2 tablespoons water; brush over dough being careful not to get it on the eggs, if you do, they can be lightly scrubbed after baking.

Bake 350°F for 30-35 minutes or until done.

Remove from sheet and cool on wire rack. Brush eggs with food coloring being careful not to get any on dough.

Drizzle orange icing over all. Makes 2 Nest Breads.

## Orange Icing

| | |
|---|---|
| 2 | cups powdered sugar or powdered sucanat with honey |
| ¼ | cup orange juice |
| ½ | tablespoons orange oil |

Mix together well and drizzle over Easter Egg Nest Bread.

# Pumpkin Bread Pudding

- 5 cups cubed bread
- 2 cups milk – any variety, my favorite is almond
- 3 eggs
- 1 cup maple syrup (option ¾ cup)
- 16 ounces pumpkin puree, either homemade or canned
- 1 cup cranberries
- 3 tablespoons melted butter
- 1 teaspoon cinnamon
- ½ teaspoon nutmeg
- ½ teaspoon ginger
- 1 teaspoon vanilla
- Cinnamon/sucanat mix for topping

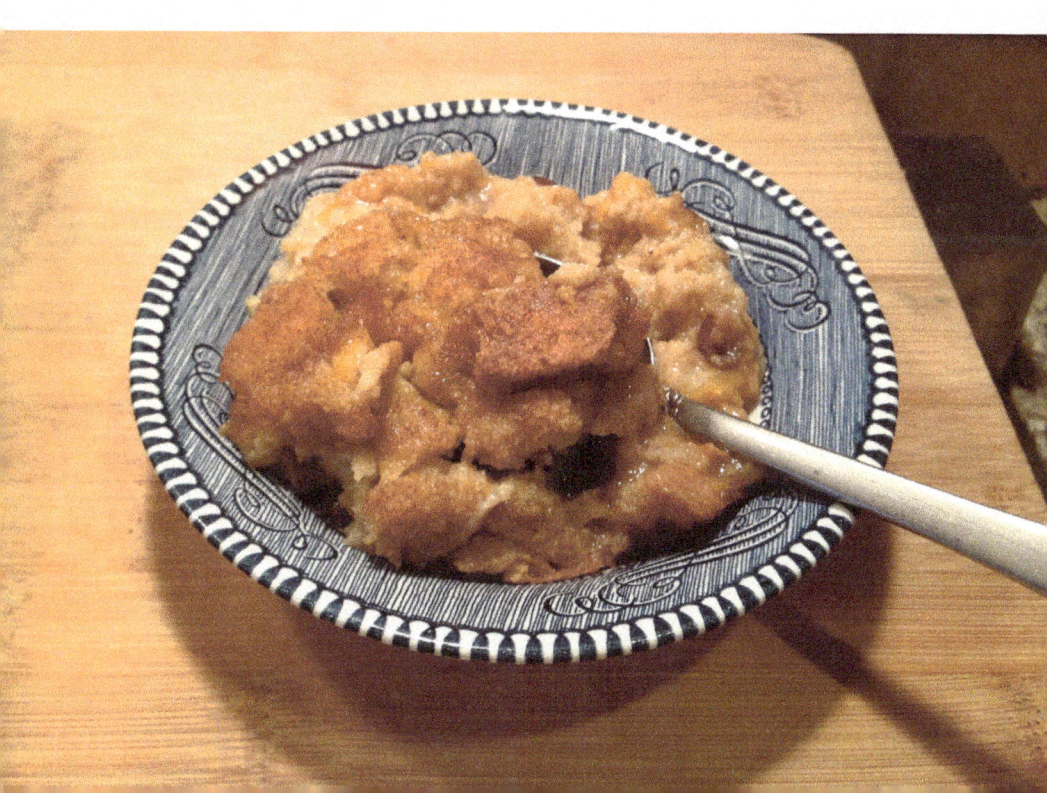

Butter an 11 x 7 baking dish

Preheat oven 350°F.

Combine milk and bread cubes and let sit.

In separate bowl combine eggs, syrup, pumpkin, cranberries, melted butter, spices, and vanilla.

Pour over soaked bread.

Pour combined mixtures into prepared baking dish and sprinkle top with cinnamon/sucanat mix.

Bake 45-60 minutes until firm and set.

Delicious as is or top with vanilla yogurt or ice cream.

# Spicy Holiday Orange-Cranberry Bread

Inspired from *Wildflour* by Denise Fidler

Knead into enough dough for 1 loaf until soft and pliable 3-4 tablespoon gluten- to lighten the loaf

### Then Add:

| | |
|---|---|
| 1 | tablespoon orange oil |
| | Rind of 1-2 organic oranges chopped fine |
| 1½ | cups dried cherries or cranberries |
| 1 | cup chopped pecans |
| ½ | teaspoon cinnamon |
| ½ | teaspoon nutmeg |
| ½ | teaspoon cloves |

Bake at 350°F for 30-35 minutes.

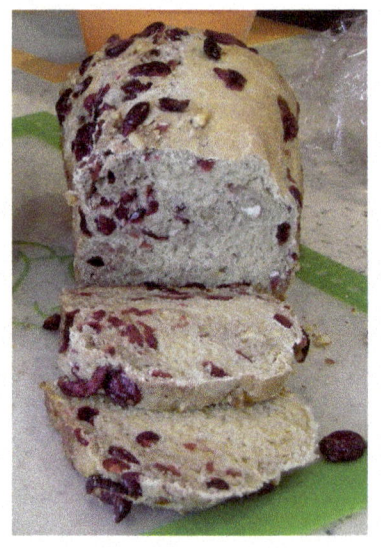

**Baking Note:** Rehydrate the cranberries for 30 minutes in warm apple juice. Drain and add to bread for a more delicious chewy texture.

An extra egg may be added to quick breads such as cornbread or banana bread to help it rise a little higher.

## Sweet Potato Biscuits

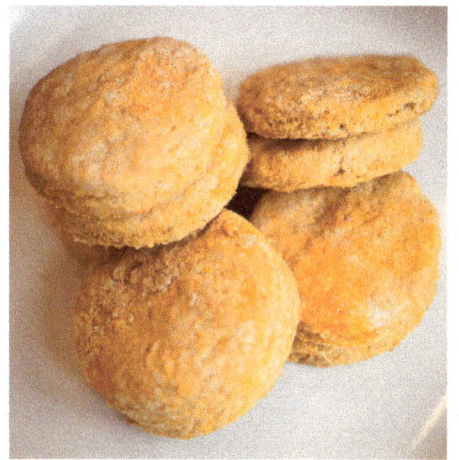

| 1   | cup freshly milled flour |
| --- | --- |
| 3   | teaspoons baking powder |
| 2   | teaspoons sucanat |
| 1   | teaspoon salt |
| 2   | tablespoons butter |
| ¾   | cup mashed sweet potatoes |
| ¼   | cup almond milk |

Preheat oven to 400°F.

In medium bowl, stir together the flour, baking powder, sucanat and salt. Add cold butter by cutting in until pieces of butter are small pea size or smaller. Mix in the sweet potatoes and enough of the milk to make a soft dough.

Turn dough out onto a floured surface, and roll or pat out to ½ inch thickness. Cut into circles using a biscuit cutter or drinking glass. Place biscuits 1 inch apart onto a greased baking sheet.

Bake for 12 – 15 minutes in the preheated oven or until golden brown.

# *My Kitchen Prayer for You*

*I pray your home is always filled with
the daily bread that only Jesus can give.
I pray your kitchen is always blessed with the
aroma of fresh milled homemade bread.
I pray you are always SATISFIED in Him.
God's Blessing's to you and your family,*

Annette Reeder

## About the author, Annette Reeder:

Annette is the founder of **The Biblical Nutritionist** and Designed Healthy Living. She is the author of over 10 published books including *Healthy Treasures Cookbook* and *Treasures of Healthy Living Bible Study*. Annette's education is not limited to her Bachelor's degree in Nutrition and diploma 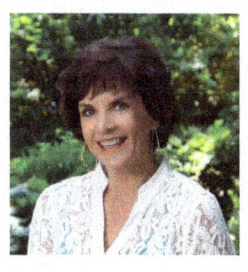 studies in Biblical Studies from Liberty University. She has numerous certifications in Metabolic Balance, Practical Nutrition, and National Speakers Association. She is a professional member of American Society of Nutrition and National Association Nutrition Professionals.

Annette considers her greatest training being a wife and mother who had to transform her family's meals from culturally correct to SATISFIED and blessed.

Annette is sought by churches to lead **Flavor of Grace Conferences** and as guidance to setting up Biblical Wellness Ministry in churches. She is a lead nutrition consultant for ministry professionals and missionaries. Her most favorite ministry desire is to share the Real Bread through cooking classes.

To secure Annette Reeder for your church visit her website for more information: www.TheBiblicalNutritionist.com. Personal consultations are available by appointment for assistance forming a biblical nutrition health plan.

## Bosch Attachments

Check www.TheBiblicalNutritionist.com for latest specials.

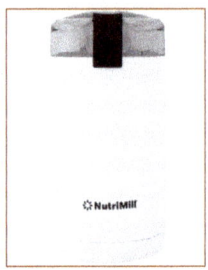
Mini Mill The perfect mini mill for seeds, herbs and chocolate.

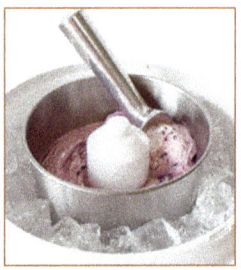
Ice Cream Maker

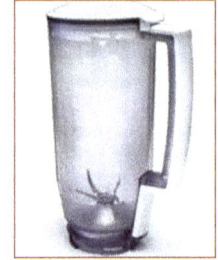
Bosch Blender

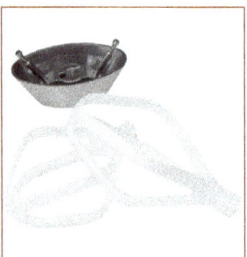
Cookie Paddles with Metal Drive

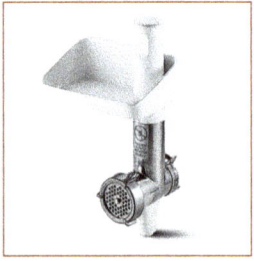
Meat & Food Grinder

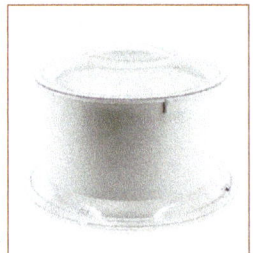
Pastry Sifter

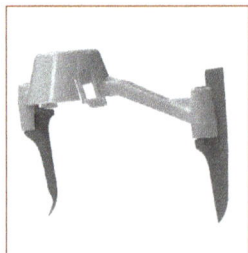
Bosch Bowl Scraper

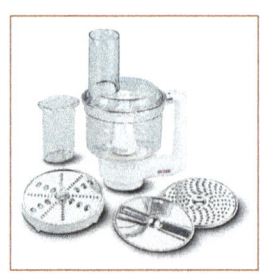
Food Processor for Bosch

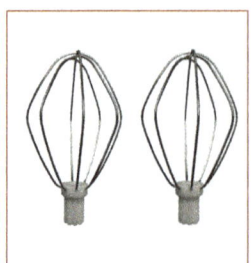
Batter Whisks

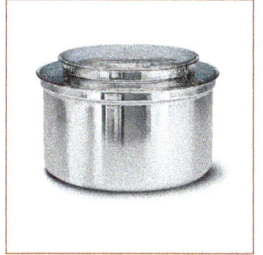 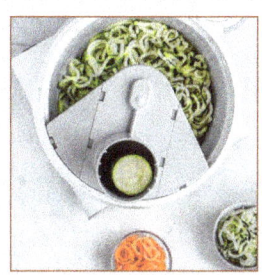 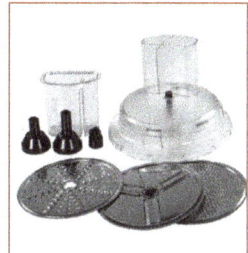

Stainless Steel Bowl for Bosch Mixer    Spiralizer    Large Slicer Shredder for Bosch Universal

## Thank You

For choosing The Biblical Nutritionist for these purchases.

It has been our joy to spend these hours with you teaching the foundation of health.

All sale profits help fund this ministry.

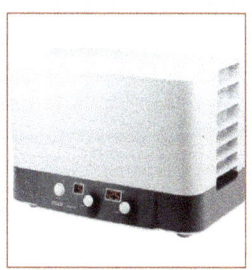

Filter – Pro Dehydrator

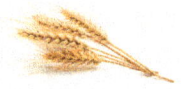

*Basic Bread Tips*

# 12 Tips For Perfect Bread

- Use instant yeast or professional yeast such as SAF. This may be added with dry ingredients and does not need to be dissolved in water.

- Store yeast in an airtight container and refrigerate or freeze to maintain freshness.

- When a recipe calls for oil and honey, put oil in measuring cup first and then honey. This allows honey to slide out more easily.

- When dough is kneaded properly, you should be able to slowly stretch a small piece into a thin windowpane, thin enough to see light through. If it tears, you may need to knead longer. Start counting kneading time as soon as you have added the last of the flour.

- It is always best to stop kneading early, rather than to over knead. Typical kneading time for whole wheat bread is 6-8 minutes, using speed 2 on the Bosch.

- To test if the dough has risen to double in size, press finger lightly and quickly into dough. If indentation springs back, let rise additional time; if indentation remains or comes back slowly, the dough has risen enough.

- Using a meat thermometer is extremely helpful in determining when the bread is done. Wheat bread is done at 190°F.
- If bread cracks on the sides, the dough has not risen long enough or too much dough has been put in the pan.
- When using craisins or raisins in baking, soften by placing in a small bowl and covering with warm juice or water to plump. Soak for 10-15 minutes.
- When baking sweet breads or braided filled breads, it may be necessary to tent the top with foil the last 5-10 minutes to avoid over browning.
- Do not over mix batters for cakes, muffins, or cookies. It causes gluten development and can make baked goods tough.
- For slicing cinnamon rolls or pizza rolls, use dental floss to cut dough.

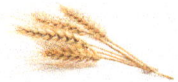

# Ingredients to Know

**Yeast** – there are several types of yeast:

> Old fashioned cake yeast – available in the dairy section – has a very short shelf life

> Active dry yeast – is dormant until it comes in contact with warm liquid, and then is brought back to life. Expiration date is longer than the cake yeast.

> Rapid rise – or quick rise – will typically allow your dough to rise in half the amount of time.

> Instant – such as SAF – is a professional brand that has been made available to the public. Very potent, greater tolerance to temperatures ranging from cool to hot. Contains live cells, you can use less and it can be added directly to the flour. Once opened it has a 1 year storage time in the freezer or 6 months in the refrigerator. Unopened it will last a long time if kept cool and dry. Stores well in a mason jar.

**Sourdough** – contains natural wild yeast from the air and no additional commercial yeast is necessary when using a pure sourdough recipe. Great for those allergic to commercial yeast.

**Dough Enhancer** – contains vitamin c, lecithin, and whey powder. Ingredients may vary depending on which brand you use. Create a favorable environment for the yeast to thrive thus creating higher rising, softer and fluffier bread. It also helps to extend the shelf life due to the lecithin. This can be used in pancakes, muffins, waffles, and more.

**Vital Gluten** – consists of gluten protein that creates strength and stability when added to the dough. This is especially helpful when using low gluten flour or adding additional ingredients such as nuts, grains, or seeds to the bread. It helps to lighten the loaf. Generally add 1 tablespoon of gluten per cup of flour. This is especially helpful when using a bread machine for a high rise and lighter bread.

**Sweetener** – Honey is the favorite – it helps to preserve the loaf and gives it a wonderful flavor. Sucanat, molasses, maple syrup, and sorghum may be used. Some French Bread does not require a sweetener.

**Salt** – helps to control the yeast and enhance the flavor of the bread. Most salt, including sea salt is heat treated and contains sugar and or aluminum as an anticaking agent. I prefer to use Real Salt™ because it is mined from the earth and has not been heat-treated, and still contains minerals.

**Fat/oil**– this is an optional ingredient for bread although it helps to preserve the loaf longer. Some bread such as French and sourdough do not use oils. Extra virgin olive oil is the healthiest choice but a good cold pressed or expeller pressed safflower, sunflower or canola oil works great, too.

**Lecithin** is granular or liquid or powdered; all forms help to preserve the freshness. The general rule of thumb to add lecithin to bread is to replace oil with 1 tablespoon per loaf or add in addition to oil if desired.

**Buttermilk** – creates a tender crumb and adds nutrition

**Potato water or** mashed potatoes- help to create a softer and fluffier loaf that stays fresher longer.

**Eggs** – add extra protein and help to preserve the loaf longer due to the lecithin in the egg.

**Vitamin C** – helps to prevent gluten strands from weakening and will help the bread to rise higher. A pinch is all you need.

**Pans** –I use a bread pan that is narrower at the bottom and wider at the top. This causes a natural rise and beautiful loaf.

**Oiling** – Use butter, nonstick spray or make your own: 2/3 cup any oil to 1/3 cup liquid lecithin stored in a jar at room temperature makes the perfect nonstick coating. Your bread should tumble right out of the pans.

**Dough additions-** If you want to add oats, grain, raisins, nuts, seeds, etc. then knead them into the dough at the end of the kneading time.

After the dough has risen, brush tops of loaves with beaten egg or egg whites and sprinkle with nuts, seeds, cracked grain, or oats on top. If you add fruits inside your bread it may require a longer baking time.

**Liquids** – you may use water, milk, buttermilk, fruit juice, or broths.

**Sponge method** – this method allows a more developed flavor without weakening the gluten. Mix your wet ingredients with some of the flour and yeast and blend slightly. Let it sit until double and then add remaining ingredients. Usually takes 20 minutes.

*Satisfied*

# Bread Cooking Helps

## *Baking*

Always be sure to have oven preheated and HOT! General rule of thumb is 350°F for 30-35 minutes when using a 1½ pound pan. Bread should be golden brown and hollow sound when thumped. Glass pans tend to over-bake and brown too quickly.

Stainless steel takes a little longer to brown. Aluminum, tin and nonstick pans seem to bake the tastiest. Don't worry about over-baked bread; it is very forgiving and will usually taste very good the first day.

All breads leftover or over browned make delicious bread crumbs and croutons. Never waste bread!

## *Cooking*

Remove bread from pans and cool on wire racks. If you are like me and want to cut into it immediately then expect a squished loaf. Waiting 15 minutes, although a test for your cravings will be the trick to keep the shape and still enjoy.

## *Freezing Baked Bread and Dough*

If stored in a heavy duty freezer bag (sold on our website), baked bread freezes very well. Use frozen bread within one month.

Frozen bread can be taken out of the freezer and allowed to thaw. Then bake in the oven for 10 minutes at 350°F. This will make it taste like you just baked it the first time.

**Refresh a stale loaf** – preheat oven to 350°F and place bread in a wet brown paper bag and bake for 5-10 minutes. My baking friend Denise Fidler shared this tip and says you will be surprised at the difference this makes!

**Slicing** – use a serrated knife for the best slices and never slice bread when it's piping hot or it will squish.

# (Endnotes)

1. Accessed 1/17/17 http://sustainableseedco.com/heirloom-grain-seed/wheat-seed/emmer-wheat-seed.html
2. Phytic Acid in Bread, Grains and Beans https://thebiblicalnutritionist.com/Phyticacid
3. What Is The Bible Diet? https://thebiblicalnutritionist.com/BibleDiet
4. Top Home Grain Mills: Best Mills for Flour and More https://thebiblicalnutritionist.com/bestgrainmills
5. Best Places to Buy Organic Whole Grains for Grinding https://thebiblicalnutritionist.com/best-places-to-buy-bulk-grains/
6. 15 Healthy Grains and Why You Should Eat Them More https://thebiblicalnutritionist.com/healthy-grains/
7. Biblical Food Pyramid Explained: What is it and is it Still Relevant? https://thebiblicalnutritionist.com/healthy-grains/
8. Barley in the Bible https://thebiblicalnutritionist.com/barley-in-the-bible/
9. Is Wheat Bad? Wheat in the Bible & Debunking Wheat Myths https://thebiblicalnutritionist.com/wheat-in-the-bible/

www.ingramcontent.com/pod-product-compliance
Lightning Source LLC
Chambersburg PA
CBHW040325300426
44112CB00021B/2882